CHEMISTRY MADE EASY

An Illustrated Study Guide For Students To Easily
Learn Chemistry

NEDU LLC

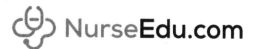

Disclaimer:

Although the author and publisher have made every effort to ensure that the information in this book was correct at press time, the author and publisher do not assume and hereby disclaim any liability to any party for any loss, damage, or disruption caused by errors or omissions, whether such errors or omissions result from negligence, accident, or any other cause.

This book is not intended as a substitute for the medical advice of physicians. The reader should regularly consult a physician in matters relating to their health, and particularly with respect to any symptoms that may require diagnosis or medical attention.

NCLEX®, NCLEX®-RN, and NCLEX®-PN are registered trademarks of the National Council of State Boards of Nursing, Inc. They hold no affiliation with this product.

Some images within this book are either royalty-free images, used under license from their respective copyright holders, or images that are in the public domain.

ISBN: 978-1-952914-05-8

FREE BONUS

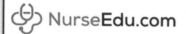

Mnemonics LAB VALUES CHEATSHEET

Explore Mnemonics Used in Nursing School & Most Commonly Found on The NCLEX.

FREE Download – Just Visit:

NurseEdu.com/bonus

TABLE OF CONTENTS

SECTION 1:
INTRODUCTION

Chemistry is a huge topic; some students spend their entire college careers studying each and every aspect of it. There are many subtopics in the study of chemistry that are woven together to create an image of what we know about atoms, molecules, and chemical reactions. There are probably millions of different chemical reactions out there. As there are currently 118 elements in the periodic table, the possibilities in the numbers and types of molecules out there are endless.

You probably don't have four years of college to devote to studying chemistry. You may not even have a semester to cram in what you need to know. No worries! This book has you covered. You will surely not be a chemistry newbie after reading this, even as you will not be able to get a chemist job anytime soon. No matter; it's probably not a job you aspire to have, anyway.

In this book, you will learn that chemistry is about matter. You can break matter down a great deal—all the way down to molecules, atoms, and subatomic particles. The smaller the matter, the weirder it gets because none of these aspects of matter can be seen under a microscope, and some are nothing more than a mathematical idea (and not a *real* thing). Don't worry; none of this is Greek, and you'll soon feel like a pro as you come to understand the language of chemistry. Let's start with the easy parts first then work our way up to more complex aspects of this fascinating (yes, really!) topic.

CHAPTER 1:

MATTER AND MEASUREMENTS
IN CHEMISTRY

You may already know what matter is and what it's made of. However, way back in the day, Empedocles (a pre-Socratic Greek who lived around 450 BC), thought he knew matter, too. He said that matter was made of one of four elements. These were air, fire, earth, and water. Most people believed this as well, until relatively recently.

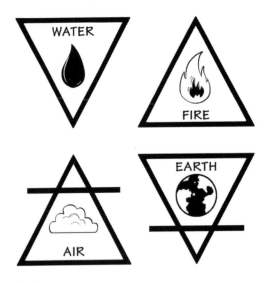

Even before Empedocles, the Greek philosophers knew of the four elements but thought only one of these was the *main* element and that the others were mostly secondary. You now know most likely that these guys had it all wrong.

Democrates in 400 BC and others had a better idea. He believed that matter was only made of two things: 1) lots of empty space and 2) tiny particles he called atoms or "atomos, " which could not be divided. In Greek, the word *atomos* means indivisible. You can see where the modern word *atom* came from! Despite being pretty close to correct about matter, Democrates was largely ignored in favor of the earlier concepts on what matter was made from.

Others (much later on) revisited this novel idea. Robert Boyle was one of these more modern-day scientists. He published a paper in 1861 where he said that an element is made of atoms that cannot be broken down under any circumstances. This put to rest the idea of four main elements. You'll see he was mostly right, too, but couldn't then have known much about atom-splitting bombs.

Boyle didn't get much credit for his work. John Dalton must have had a better publicity agent because he is credited with what we now know is modern atomic theory. In reality, he was first, after all, having published his atomic theory in 1803. He had some great theories on atoms. These include:

1. All matter is made from atoms. Atoms cannot be destroyed or divided.
2. All atoms of the same element will also be the same or identical.
3. Atoms from different elements have different properties and different atomic weights.
4. One can combine different atoms in whole numbers to create a new molecule.
5. If a compound decomposes, all atoms can be recovered as they can't be destroyed.
6. Atoms cannot be created from nothing.
7. Chemical reactions just rearrange atoms in molecules. They do not make new atoms.

Mass or matter is always conserved in any isolated system. This is a fact best explained by the Law of Conservation of Mass. This idea also came from the Greeks, who believed that all the matter in the universe is neither created nor destroyed. Antoine Lavoisier described this principle in 1789. This statement is absolutely true when you maintain a closed system.

Think about it: *If you mix two substances in solution and one of the end products is a gaseous substance, you might doubt the Law of Conservation of Matter if you weigh the products left in the reaction flask. The end products will not have the same weight as the beginning substrates. This is because, unless you close the system up and keep the gas inside the "system," the gas escapes and isn't counted. Anytime you do a chemical reaction, you need to think about what might leave the system afterward for any reason.*

Einstein extended the law of conservation of mass to add energy into the equation. Energy and mass are both parts of any reaction system. Because of this, the total energy plus the mass in a system are always constant. This gets a little more complicated, so most chemists ignore the energy aspect of a reaction. This is because most lab-table chemical reactions don't make much energy.

Joseph Proust got a law named after himself in the early 1800s by conducting experiments on the composition of simple molecules. He realized that all compounds are made by mixing elements in fixed proportions. The molecule of carbon dioxide, or CO_2, for example, will always be made from a single atom of carbon and two of oxygen. He went further by noting that the mass of CO_2 in a system will be fixed in how much of it is carbon and how much is oxygen. Two oxygen atoms have an atomic mass of 16 x 2 or 32, while one carbon atom has an atomic mass of 12. The ratio then is 12:32 or about 3:8 (by weight).

Classification of Matter

Now that you know what matter is (atoms with a lot of space around them), you should be curious about some of the details that define matter more clearly. An enclosed box with a kilogram of carbon dioxide gas and a block of dry ice are both matter, but you would never call them the same thing. Chemically, they are the same, but nothing else about them would indicate this.

Suppose you got a mystery box with matter in it, without knowing what it was. Without being able to name the substance or matter in the box, how would you describe it to others? How would you go about this descriptive process, and what properties would you talk about in telling others about it? Let's look at ways chemists talk about the different properties of matter; these would be terms you would use to describe your mystery matter.

Start with recognizing two separate categories of *properties of matter*. One of these is its physical properties. You don't have to do much to identify these besides measure, weigh, and observe. Physical properties are also divided into two segments: 1) those unrelated to how much of the substance you have (intensive physical properties) and 2) those dependent on how much you have (extensive physical properties). They break down like this:

Intensive Physical Properties	Extensive Physical Properties	Chemical Properties
Color	Mass	Reaction with acids
Density	Volume	Response to air exposure
Melting point	Length	Reaction with bases
Boiling point	Shape	Reaction in water
Conductivity		Reaction in other substances
Malleability		

With your mystery matter, start with the easy things:

Extensive Physical Properties

These are obvious and just involve a few measuring tools, like a scale and measuring tape.

1. **How much does it weigh?** Measure this in grams or kilograms, generally.
2. **What volume is it?** Measure this in cubic centimeters (millimeters) or another convenient measurement, remembering that volume is height x width x depth.
3. **What length is it?** Obviously, this works best with solids. Get its dimensions in centimeters or meters on all possible sides, knowing it may not be a nice rectangular shape. A ball of something would still be measured using the volume of a sphere: $V = 4/3\,\pi r^3$.
4. **What shape is it?** Be creative. If you think it's a shape you can identify, go ahead and call it as you see it. Otherwise, take your best guess on what shape it is (for solids, obviously).

Intensive Physical Properties

Some of these are easy, like color and malleability. FYI: Malleability means whether or not you can flatten the substance out. Here are a few others:

1. **How dense is it?** Density is determined by weighing it and getting its volume. The density of a liquid, for example, is often in grams/milliliters. You get this by taking the weight and dividing it by the volume. You can plainly see without measuring, however,

that an oily substance is less dense than water, just by mixing the two and seeing if the density is different:

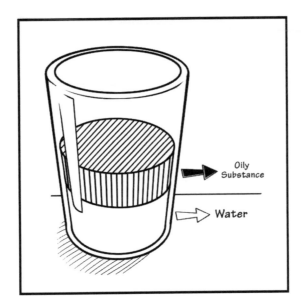

2. **What is its melting point?** Melting point and freezing point are the same things. As we will discuss soon, the melting point is best found by melting a solid first and sticking a thermometer in it. Then cool it down and determine when it freezes again. If you can't do that, it's harder to measure. You need to heat up the solid and then determine the temperature in the system when it melts.

3. **What is its boiling point?** Again, the boiling point is the same as the condensation temperature. Both of these measure the liquid-to-gas phase change of a substance. You would do the same thing as with the melting point. Put a thermometer in a liquid and add heat. Then find out when it begins to boil. This is your boiling point.

4. **Does it have conductivity?** This is a substance that conducts electricity. You will need to have two electrodes (be creative about this). Then measure if any electricity flows from one electrode to another. If yes, it conducts electricity. This is how it's done in liquids:

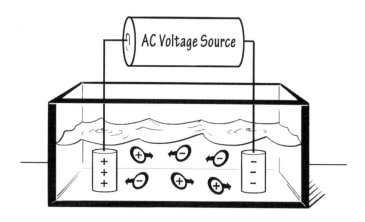

Chemical Properties

These are more sophisticated and depend on knowing much more about chemistry (like what acids and bases are, for example) than you are expected to know yet. The fact is that most matter will respond in some way to another bit of matter. The sky is the limit here. You can describe what a substance dissolves in (or doesn't dissolve in). Many metals will react in acid...try putting some zinc metal in hydrochloric acid, but beware of the hydrogen gas it gives off.

> **Don't try this at home!** Obviously, you can put as much sodium chloride (NaCl or table salt) in water without much risk. Try this with sodium metal, however, and the results are remarkable (and dangerous!). Sodium metal comes packed in oil to keep it away from moisture. Throw it in water and watch it violently explode to make sodium hydroxide and a lot of hydrogen gas! Definitely not something to try at home...

You can only do so much when describing chemical properties. If you tried to describe a chunk of sodium metal by putting the whole thing in water, you'd have a solution of sodium hydroxide and no more sodium metal to experiment with. Still, a few judicious experiments might clue you in as to the properties of the matter you have.

Phases of Matter

If you think this is an easy section, you might want to consider this: is water (H2O) a solid, liquid, or gas? The answer is obvious, which is that *it all depends*. But what does it depend on? Temperature? Yes, partly, but you'll see it's more complicated than that. Let's start with getting clear on what the different phases of matter look like:

- **Solids**—these are substances that do not need a container to hold their shape. The molecules tend to be fixed in space and are generally tightly packed. While they cannot move freely in relation to one another, molecules in solid form will still vibrate.

  Many solids are crystalline, meaning they are packed tightly in an ordered shape. The crystals can be unique to a substance or can change in the same substance, depending on pressure and temperature issues.

  This is how crystalline and amorphous solids might look:

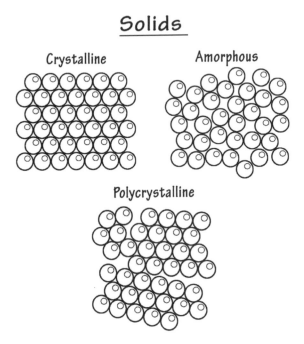

- **Gases**—these are substances that must be fully contained in a container with sides everywhere, although gravity can hold some gases in a collection without borders. There are intermolecular interactions, but these are small, so the molecules in gaseous form move freely. Gaseous molecules move very fast compared to solid and liquid molecules; their kinetic energy (tendency to be zippy, that is) overrides most of the forces between any two gaseous molecules. Gases have large spaces between the tiny molecules.

Gases

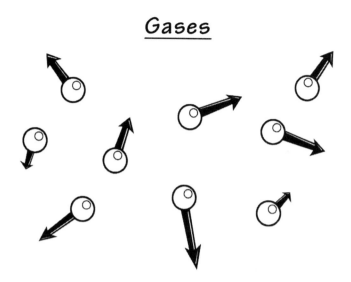

- **Liquids**—these will flow and cannot maintain a definite shape unless held in a container on most of its sides. The molecules move freely but stay within the boundaries of the volume they reside in. The volume of a liquid always stays the same, but the shape does not. There are some intermolecular forces important in liquids, but these are not so great at keeping the molecules fixed in space. Most of the time, a liquid will be less dense than its corresponding solid (water, aka ice, is a notable exception).

Liquids

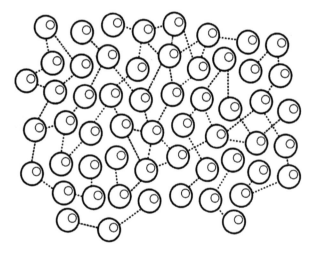

There are several phases of matter you won't encounter often. One of these is called *plasma*. Plasma is interesting. It's the gaseous stuff the sun gives off of its surface. While it is gaseous, plasma differs from a true gas in that it is a mixture of charged molecules that interact with one another and that generate long-range magnetic and electric fields. One glob of plasma would be electrically neutral, but a lot of electrical interactions are going on within the glob.

Trick question: Is glass a liquid or solid? The real answer is neither. It is referred to as an amorphous solid because the molecules are not in any orderly structure (like a crystal lattice). Over time, the molecules do move, but it takes billions of years for a glass (silicate) molecule to travel even a small distance.

Phase Changes

Obviously, matter can change phases. Some of these you know well, such as melting, freezing, and boiling. These are not all the possible choices, however. You'll see just how many choices a chunk of matter can go through.

The reality is that no matter is anything but solid at absolute zero (-273 degrees Celsius). Even helium gas would be solid at that temperature. In the same way, at high enough temperatures, all things will be liquid. To be certain, it is impossible to get absolute zero, and, in order to make gaseous iron, you'd need to reach 2861 degrees Celsius. Still, you get the idea...

Next order of business: is a phase change all about raising or lowering the temperature of matter? Not in the slightest. Pressure has a lot to do with it. If you add enough pressure to something, you can change its phase from gas to liquid to solid without cooling anything at all.

When it comes to phase changes, these are the ones you should know:

- **Freezing**—going from a liquid to a solid by removing thermal heat or cooling a substance (generally, the pressure remains the same).
- **Melting**—going from a solid to a liquid by adding heat to a substance (molecules vibrate from the added energy and reach a liquid state).
- **Sublimation**—going from a solid to a gas, skipping the liquid stage. You will see sublimation when you watch dry ice in a warm temperature; you will see a mist coming

off the dry ice. This is sublimation. Freeze-drying involves removing water in a vacuum, which essentially sublimates it, leaving the dried matter behind.

- **Vaporization**—going from a liquid to a gas, which can happen by boiling or allowing the liquid to evaporate. When boiling is the type of vaporization happening, heat is added to a system to give the internal energy they need to move about in gaseous form.
- **Condensation**—going from a gas to a liquid through cooling and losing molecular energy. When water vapor or humidity in the air is allowed to cool in the nighttime, dew will condense onto the grass every morning.
- **Deposition**—going from gaseous form to solid form, skipping the liquid step. When frost forms on grass or another solid surface, this is called deposition.

There is one interesting feature you'll note about phase changes. If you were to take a pan of water and start raising the temperature, it would rise steadily until it reached the boiling point of 100 degrees Celsius. It will stop there, however, as the water is boiling away. Why doesn't it go any further? This is because it takes a lot of energy to go through a phase change. Energy that would normally go into raising the temperature of the system is diverted to cause the phase change. If you boiled all the water away in an enclosed space, the temperature would only rise again after the phase change was complete. It works this way for lowering or raising the temperature in a phase change situation.

This graph shows you how the phase changes of water work. You see how the temperature plateaus precisely at each phase change:

Phase Diagram

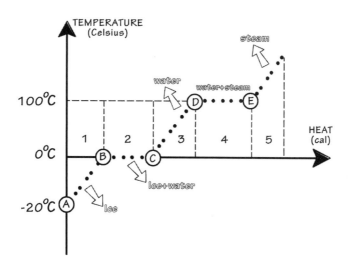

Understanding the Phase Diagram

You need to understand that pressure and temperature change when a substance goes through any phase change. You don't see this issue in your everyday surroundings because the pressure changes, but if you moved to a high altitude after living at sea level, you might see the difference. This is how it works:

The air pressure at sea level is 1 atmosphere or 760 mmHg. Water boils at this pressure at 100.0 degrees Celsius (212 degrees Fahrenheit). As you go up in altitude, the boiling point will drop. This is because the air pressure is less at higher altitudes. By the time you get to about 2500 meters in altitude or 8000 feet, the air pressure is just 0.74 atmospheres or 570 mmHg. At this altitude, you will boil water at just 94 degrees Celsius (198 degrees Fahrenheit).

This phase diagram will show you some interesting things if you stare at it for a while:

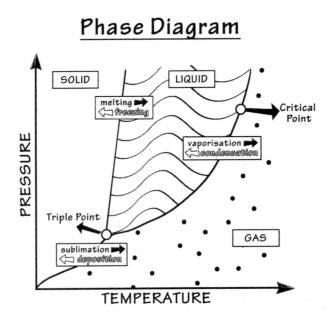

Notice how the different phases are all represented and where there are changes as you add temperature and pressure to the system. You can see where the phase changes occur. The phase boundary is the line at any given pressure and temperature that a phase change happens. The triple point is a spot on the diagram where you could technically have the solid, liquid, and gaseous forms exist in relative equilibrium.

The critical point is a no-man's-land where you just can't have liquid. Instead, you get what's called a supercritical fluid. Supercritical fluids are high-temperature, high-pressure fluids with a great deal of energy in the molecules. These fluids behave like liquids, but they also have compressibility you won't see in non-supercritical fluids.

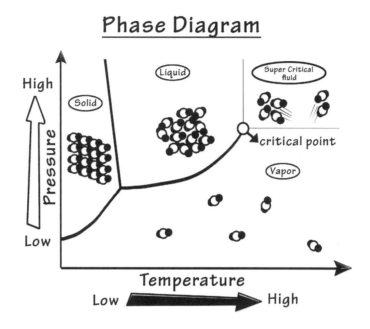

Let's Wrap This Up

Everything you can think of is made from matter (except a pure vacuum, which is hard to achieve). We've come a long way from having four elements to a giant periodic table with numerous elements and a much clearer explanation of what matter is all about.

You now know how to describe the properties of matter and the different phases of matter. Phase changes happen in all elements and molecules to some degree, even though it is very hard to boil most metallic substances. You should study the phase diagram of water as an example of what they look like under different pressure and temperature conditions.

CHAPTER 2:

IMPORTANT NUMBERS
AND TERMS TO KNOW

You may have read terms so far that have confused you. Chemistry, (like all other branches of science) has its own lingo. If you do not know this language, you will struggle from the beginning to get the concepts. This chapter is an attempt to get you started on the right foot.

There are a few things you should understand that are a bit more boring. They have to do with how scientific information is presented. You do not need to memorize it all; instead, bookmark this page so you can refer back to it when making calculations or trying to understand why chemical symbols and equations look the way they do. Ready?

The Periodic Table

You will learn more about the periodic table than you might think possible in Chapter 4. Until then, you should take a look at this one and stare in awe over how complex it is. You will soon know why it is in such a funny shape and what it all means. For now, use this table for any calculations in this chapter:

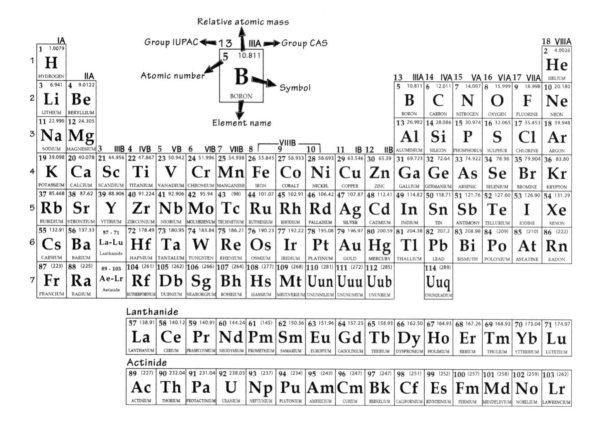

Terms to Know

There are some words used all the time in chemistry. This is the lingo of this branch of science. If you understand what they mean, you will breeze through this book without difficulty.

- **Matter**—anything in the universe that has mass (weight) and takes up space.
- **Atom**—the simplest piece of matter in the universe. For all practical purposes in chemistry, atoms cannot be split.

- **Element**—any unique substance with atoms that are generally all the same size. Elements are specifically identified by their atomic size.
- **Periodic table**—a table of all of the elements, along with the atomic weights. Use the periodic table (which is covered later) to learn about the known properties of the different elements. There is a reason why the periodic table looks like it does.
- **Nucleus**—the central part of an atom, made of neutrons and protons (see image).

Atom Particles

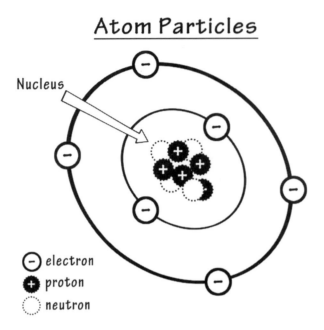

- ⊖ electron
- ⊕ proton
- ◌ neutron

- **Proton**—a positively-charged particle in the center of the atom.
- **Neutron**—a neutrally-charged particle in the center of the atom. Essentially, only neutrons and protons add to the weight of an atom. Most atoms have equal numbers of protons and neutrons (but this isn't universally true, as you will see).
- **Electrons**—a negatively -harged particle in an atom that exists on the periphery of an atom. Its mass is negligible. The number of electrons in an atom is different for each element and doesn't ever change as long as the atom is neutral (not charged in any way).
- **Isotope**—any atom that has the same number of protons and electrons as another atom but differs in mass because it has a different number of neutrally-charged neutrons in the atomic nucleus. Most isotopes have differing numbers of protons and neutrons and aren't as commonly seen in nature as the natural atom of any element (which has equal numbers of protons and neutrons).
- **Ion**—an atom that is charged because it has lost or gained electrons.

- **Anion**—a negatively-charged ion that has gained at least one electron. A molecule (more than one atom together) can also be an ion as a single group. $H_2PO_4^-$ is a type of ion made from more than one type of element. Its name is dihydrogen phosphate.

- **Cation**—a positively-charged ion that has lost at least one electron. A cation can also be a small molecule that is charged as a single group. NH_4^+, for example, is a positively-charged cation called an ammonium ion.

- **Isotope**—an element with at least one extra neutron added or missing, slightly affecting the actual atomic mass of an element you'll see in the periodic table (more on that later).

- **Atomic mass**—the mass of an atom in kilograms or Daltons or atomic mass units. A Dalton is an odd measurement; it is defined as $1/12$ of the mass of one carbon-12 atom. One Dalton is equal to 1.66×10^{-27} kilograms (give or take a few milligrams).

- **Molecule**—this describes any grouping of atoms that may contain the same or different elements. A molecule can be as simple as H_2 (which is hydrogen gas) or as complex as a protein with thousands of atoms in it.

There are many more chemistry terms you will learn; these are simply the basics. Once you learn these simple terms, the text you read from now on will be far more understandable.

International System of Units

The different units used in science can be dizzying. You can measure weight in pounds, grams, kilograms, or stones (depending on where you live and what you're used to). You can measure temperature in Fahrenheit, Kelvin, or Celsius. This problem makes it complicated to figure out what a person is talking about, especially if they aren't consistent in their message.

The issue was partly laid to rest in 1960 when a conference was held by the General Conference on Weights and Measures (CGWM). This was the 11th conference held by the group, first begun in 1875, in order to keep measurements as uniform as possible. They adopted the SI system or the International System of Units. The group laid out which units were to be standard throughout the world.

Most of these units are used in chemistry (and this book will use them as much as possible). Frankly, it's hard not to mess up because there are a lot of nonstandard units of measure (such as the Dalton and mmHg for air pressure). Still, you should try to stick with this metric unit-based system as much as you can.

This table shows you some of these SI units you should use:

Measurement	SI Unit	Abbreviation	Measurement	SI Unit	Abbreviation
Length	Meter	m	Angle	Radian	Rad
Mass	Kilogram	kg	Frequency	Hertz	Hz
Time	second	s	Force	Newton	N
Current	Ampere	A	Pressure	Pascal	Pa
Temperature	Kelvin	K	Energy/work	Joule	J
Amount	Mole	mol	Power	Watt	W
Area	Square meter	m^2	Charge	Coulomb	C
Volume	Cubic meter	m^3	Electric force	Volt	V
Velocity	Meter per sec	m/s	Resistance	Ohm	Ω
Acceleration	Meter/sec²	m/s^2	Radiation	Gray	Gy
Mass density	Kilogram/m³	kg/m^3	Magnetic flux	Weber	Wb

You need to remember your basic knowledge of the metric system and know what it means to add prefixes to some of these (or take them away). This knowledge will lead to terms like centimeter, millimeter, grams, milliliters, etc. These are terms you might use more often in chemistry than you will the actual SI unit listed in the table.

Scientific Notation

This part is relatively easy, but if you haven't done it in a while, you will need to refresh yourself. Remember that numbers in science can be very large or very small. It means you need some way to express one quadrillion or more of something. You could write 1,000,000,000,000,000, but that would be cumbersome. Instead, using scientific notation, you would write it in one of several ways:

- 1×10^{15}
- $1 \times 10^{\wedge}15$

- 1e15

You should also know these things apply to very small numbers. Instead of writing 0.00001, you will write it in scientific notation to indicate any of these things:

- 1×10^{-5}

- $1 \times 10^{\wedge}-5$

- 1e-5

Makes sense, right?

Now that you understand this, you should know some terminology used in chemistry specifically. When you look at the periodic table, you will see a dizzying number of abbreviations for the different elements. This may be hard to believe, but you will need to memorize a lot of these—at least the first four rows, or *periods*, and a few in the fifth period. There is no other way around it. Get some flashcards (or make some), so you can get the abbreviations for the elements memorized quickly.

The other thing you'll want to have clear is how molecules are written. If you are reading this book and come across an abbreviation for a molecule, you should know what it means. Here are a few ways to write molecules:

- **NaCl**—the formula for sodium chloride (table salt). Na is the abbreviation for sodium, and Cl is the abbreviation for chloride. There are no numbers associated with this formula because the molecule consists of a single atom of sodium and a single atom of chloride. Easy, right?

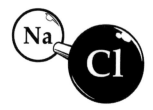

- **H2 or H_2**—the molecular formula for hydrogen gas. H is the abbreviation for hydrogen. The number 2 is used to mean that the molecule contains 2 of these hydrogen atoms.

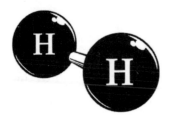

- **C6H12O6 or $C_6H_{12}O_6$**—can mean a lot of things, but in organic chemistry, a six-carbon sugar like glucose. It is a significant abbreviation that gives you no clue about what the molecule really looks like. Here is what glucose generally looks like if you could see it up close:

- **KOH**—the formula for potassium hydroxide. K is the abbreviation for potassium, and OH is the abbreviation for hydroxide. You will find out later that it isn't written OHK because potassium is positively charged and OH is negatively charged. The positively-charged cation is always written first. When you write the potassium ion, write K+; when you write the hydroxide ion, write: OH-.

Significant Calculations used in Chemistry

These are a few things you need to understand before proceeding. If you don't understand them completely, do not worry. You should have some idea, however, what these things mean. Later on, you will master the art of doing it all yourself.

Stoichiometry

Stoichiometry is a long word used mainly in chemistry. You use this type of chemistry math to know how to balance chemical equations and figure out how much of each substance you need to use up all of the reactants (starting substances in the laboratory).

In any chemical equation, you will have reactants that undergo a chemical change to make products. An example equation looks like this:

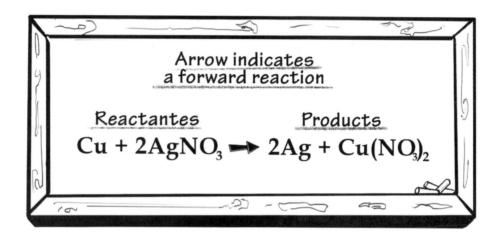

You know this is a balanced reaction because if you add the number of each molecule on each side of the arrow, the number should be equal on both sides. Just add these numbers up, and if you get equal numbers on both sides, the equation is *balanced*.

What is a Mole?

Moles are used to determine how much of a substance you have. Chemistry is great because it doesn't matter if an element is very small versus gigantic. A mole is simply the number of molecules you have. It's that easy. It's just a number.

If you really counted all the molecules you had in a flask, however, the number would be gigantic and too wieldy to work with. An Italian scientist in the early 1800s named Amadeo Avogadro worked on this issue. Later on, someone honored his work by naming a famous number after him. Avogadro's number is something you should memorize: it is the number of molecules in one mole of any molecule or element. Avogadro'*s number is 6.022 x 10²³ molecules per mole*.

If you have a mole of hydrogen gas and a mole of neon gas, they weigh differing amounts. How do you figure out how much of each gas to put in a container if you want a 50:50 mixture (by moles) of each substance? Actually, it's not hard. What you'll learn is that the periodic table shows the atomic number of each element. **This is the mass of one mole of the element in the box in the table**. It looks like this:

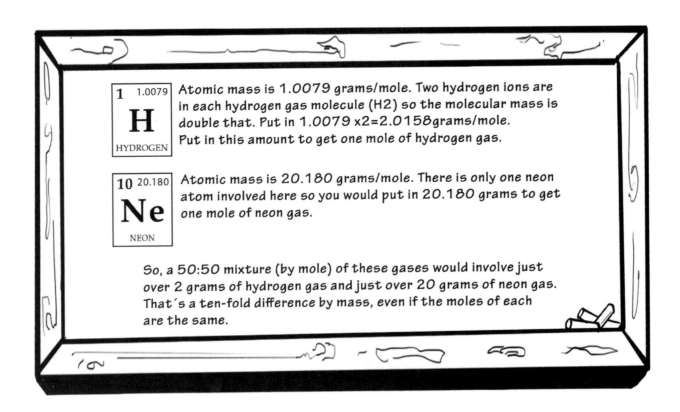

1 1.0079
H
HYDROGEN

Atomic mass is 1.0079 grams/mole. Two hydrogen ions are in each hydrogen gas molecule (H2) so the molecular mass is double that. Put in 1.0079 x2=2.0158grams/mole. Put in this amount to get one mole of hydrogen gas.

10 20.180
Ne
NEON

Atomic mass is 20.180 grams/mole. There is only one neon atom involved here so you would put in 20.180 grams to get one mole of neon gas.

So, a 50:50 mixture (by mole) of these gases would involve just over 2 grams of hydrogen gas and just over 20 grams of neon gas. That's a ten-fold difference by mass, even if the moles of each are the same.

Determining the Percent Composition by Mass of a Substance in Solution

This is basic science in action—a lot of benchwork thinking is involved. Unfortunately, much of chemistry is done in laboratories, so you should know a few basics on how to measure things. This calculation involves getting a weight percent of something in solution. The *solute* is the stuff you put in the liquid to make *a solution*. The *solvent* is the liquid you are using. Usually, the solvent is water, which is why we call it an *aqueous solution*. The term *aqueous* means *water*. So, how do we do this?

You need two things: 1) the mass of the solute (usually in grams) and 2) the mass of the solution. The tricky part is that the mass of the solution is NOT THE SAME as the mass of the solvent. Once you add the solute, the solvent becomes a solution that is heavier than it was. So, let's try this:

- Sodium chloride added is 12.0 grams
- Solvent (water) is 100 ml. The hard part is that water should weigh about 1g/ml, but it is slightly less than this at room temperature, so you will notice it weighs exactly 99.8 grams, rather than 100 grams.

Now, when you calculate your percent mass, you'll get this:

$$Percent\ mass = \frac{12.0}{12.0 + 99.8}\ x\ 100 = 10.7\ percent$$

Pay attention: You should try to use significant figures that are consistent throughout your equations. This means that when you are working with a number like 12.1 (accurate to 1/10th) and one like 14.223 (accurate to 1/1000th), you should simplify the second number to 14.2 instead (unless it is very important not to do this for some reason). Keep in mind what you are doing. If you are baking a cake, one cup could mean 1.12 cups; the cake will be fine. If you are doing a precise experiment, however, you need to know if you mean 1.0, 1.1, or 1.12. It might matter, you know?

Figuring out Molarity and Moles

Many things in chemistry are messier than you would think. What if, for example, you are told to make a 1M solution in water? This means a solution where one mole of any molecule exits in solution. How do you do this?

First, you need to know what the solute is. Let's say it's potassium bromide or KBr. How much of this stuff is a mole? The answer lies in the periodic table again. Find the molar mass on the upper righthand corner of each element (it might be below your element's abbreviation on your own table).

- Potassium—30.098—grams per mole
- Bromine—79.904 grams per mole
- Potassium bromide—30.098 + 79.904 = 110.002 grams per mole

You can probably round it to 110.0 grams per mole of the molecule (which will be a solid salt).

Now you need to put 110.0 grams of the KBr into a beaker or flask. Then, add enough water, so the total amount is 1 liter. Stir it up, and get a 1M solution (one mole/liter) containing 110.0 grams/liters of this salt. If you add exactly a liter of water to the solute, it will be slightly off because the salt will somewhat displace the water. It won't make much difference unless the concentration of solute in the solution is high, however.

Molality is a term you might hear about, too. What is the difference between molality and molarity, anyway? Just remember this:

- Molarity—this is the number of moles per liter (volume) of the _solution_.
- Molality—this is the number of moles of the solute divided by the mass in kilograms (mass and not volume) of the _solvent_.

So, it's messy. One liter of a solution of water plus the solute weighs more than a liter of water (the solvent) by itself. The molarity and molality will not be identical.

There are molarity-to-molality calculators on the internet that are very helpful. Say, for example, you have a solute in water that contains 1 mole/liter of solution (density of 997 kg/m³). Now, if that solution has KBr in it (molar mass of 110.0 grams per mole), according to these calculators, your 1M solution (molarity) will be 1.064m (the letter m is the abbreviation for molality). It is difficult to make this calculation by yourself (but not impossible), so use an online converter if you can.

Let's Wrap This Up

This chapter allowed you to dip your toes into chemistry by learning the lingo and seeing the main players (the elements in the periodic table). You need to memorize the elements and their abbreviations, and you need to know what a molecule is just by seeing the abbreviation. The number after the abbreviation is the number of atoms in the molecule. You should use this chapter as a reference, in case you forget the terms or how to balance equations (we will talk more about this later).

Now that you have a bit of chemistry knowledge, we will dive right in and learn what atoms and molecules look like up close. You will also learn more about the periodic table and chemical reactions. Step-by-step, you will feel like you understand chemistry in the most painless way possible.

SECTION 2:
THE STRUCTURE OF MATTER

This section builds upon the idea of matter being composed of atoms. We will start with the atom, which is technically unable to be broken down but is itself composed of tinier particles (electrons, protons, and neutrons). Even smaller than these are things like quarks, which are studied in quantum mechanics classes rather than traditional chemistry courses. Quarks and similar particles are fun but make no real difference in the chemistry of an atom or molecule.

Atoms associate with one another to make molecules. We will talk a lot about the periodic table and the many things you can get out of studying it. Once you understand the different properties of the elements, you'll understand why some do nothing in a chemical reaction and others are highly reactive, forming covalent or ionic bonds easily with other elements.

CHAPTER 3:

ATOMIC THEORY

Atomic theory has evolved over time—from the days of the ancient Greeks to Dalton and beyond. Two of the more common approaches to understanding what atoms might look like come from the Bohr model and the quantum mechanical model of the atom. These two models are not the same, but neither is incorrect; both have reasonable applications to the study of the atom and how it functions in chemistry.

The Bohr Model of the Atom

Before the Bohr model (which was proposed by Niels Bohr in 1913), there was the Rutherford model, first proposed by Ernest Rutherford. He had a theory about the atom that was at least partially correct. He knew there was a dense and heavy (from an atomic perspective) core in the atom; it was made of positively-charged particles he called neutrons. He believed that there were probably neutral particles called neutrons as well.

Where he got it wrong was in the action of electrons, which are the negatively-charged and extremely lightweight particles in the periphery of the atom. Rutherford thought it would make sense to have the electrons orbit the nucleus of the atom, much like the planets orbit the sun. This model, called the planetary model, was cool but entirely inaccurate.

The Bohr Model of Atom

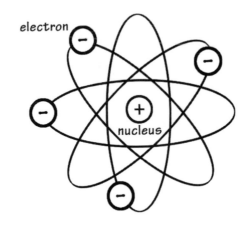

Niels Bohr had other ideas. He had an inkling of what we now know as quantum theory and used this in his description of the atom.

Quantum theory is complex, but, in simple terms, you need to think of quanta (singular is quantum) as packets of particles that can interact with one another but only in specific ways. Electrons behave more like small packets of energy and less like things you can see or touch. Rather than electrons mindlessly orbiting a nucleus, they are found in certain areas of the atom in different and specific energy states. To best understand these ideas, you need to know a few facts:

1. ***Electrons are negatively charged****. In general, *they do not like to stand near each other* (because their charges are the same and, like a magnet, positive attracts negative, but negatives repel each other).

2. ***Electrons prefer a low-energy state if possible***. Wouldn't you? The idea is that electrons will jump from one energy state to another if conditions are right, but in general, lower energy states are preferred.

3. ***Electrons should not be thought of as gliding from one place to another***. Instead, they *hop from one energy state to another*. This is a hard concept to grasp; remember, though, they are very small and don't have the mass it takes to gradually drift about. Think of hummingbirds instead that flit from place to place. They travel from flower to flower, but the in-between part is vague and hard to see.

4. ***Quantum theory applies to electrons because they are so small***. This is best explained by thinking about momentum. If you shine a light on an elephant in the dark,

for example, the photons of light don't move the elephant by shining on it. It is too big, and it would take more force than a light ray to move it. Electrons are so tiny and relatively massless ($9.10938356 \times 10^{-31}$ kilograms) that they will get bumped out of the way as soon as you *shine a light on them* to see where they are. This makes electrons unique and have properties not exactly particle-like. (We'll talk more about that later).

Bohr spent a long time studying the hydrogen atom, which is the simplest atom. He agreed with the idea of electrons orbiting the nucleus but realized they must orbit at specific levels. He felt it was a lot like how each planet has its own radius from the sun, except that electrons could jump from one orbital radius to another. This is Bohr's idea of a hydrogen atom:

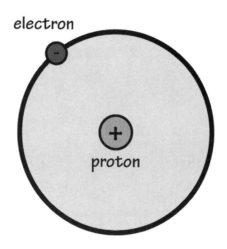

According to this model, each radius is given a whole number, or integer. The radii nearest to the nucleus get the lowest number. These also have the lowest energy states. Under certain conditions, electrons can jump from one radius to another (but not in between). As an electron jumps from one energy state to another (from a high-to-low energy state), it will give off radiation (a teeny-tiny amount, just 13.6eV or the same as one photon of light). The electromagnetic radiation given off is like a light wave that delivers light in quanta or packets of energy. This image shows you what it looks like:

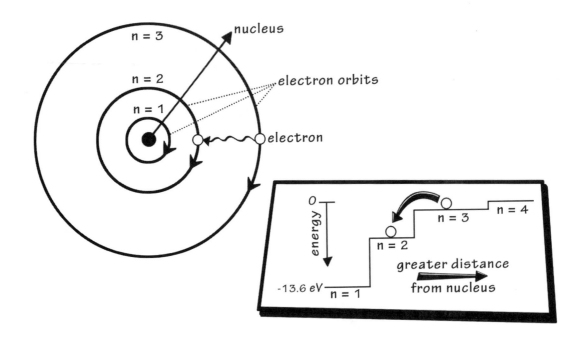

Bohr had a great idea, but it too was simple than it is in larger atoms. The hydrogen atom has just a single proton and an electron. There is essentially no interaction with other electrons within this tiny atom by itself. This why, in nature, hydrogen is seen as a diatomic gas called H_2 (two atoms of hydrogen together).

If this part seems hard to understand or maybe meaningless, you will get the idea soon. This next theory allows you to see where electrons lie in complicated (bigger) atoms and shows you how electrons help atoms form bonds to make larger molecules.

The Quantum-Mechanical Model of the Atom

Things get a little stickier when you talk about the quantum-mechanical model of the atom. One key feature of quantum mechanics is that _everything is both a particle and a wave_ (at the same time!). Everything—all large and small things in the universe—fall into this category, but the thing to remember is that big things are far more _particle_ than _wave_. The opposite is true of small things. When you get very small, like photon-sized and electron-sized things, everything gets topsy-turvy, and you need to really think of a _wave more than a particle_ with these substances.

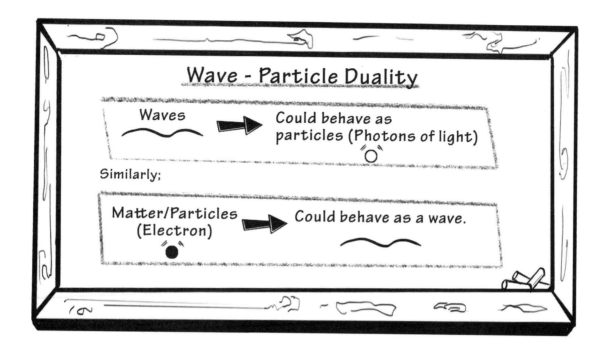

Why is this important in chemistry? Well, after some messy mathematics, the principles of quantum mechanics mean that this whole idea of circular orbits around a nucleus needs to be thrown out. You can't really expect an electron to behave so perfectly, given how small it is and how non-particle it seems to be. Instead, you need to find places around the nucleus of the atom _where it is most likely to be_. Instead of saying "an electron is here," you would say where there is a high probability of finding an electron.

Old Atomic Theories

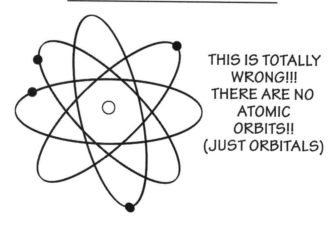

THIS IS TOTALLY WRONG!!! THERE ARE NO ATOMIC ORBITS!! (JUST ORBITALS)

So, now instead of _orbits_, we have _orbitals_. Orbitals are where it is most probable that an electron will be. It isn't always a nice circle. It's more like a cloud where you'll see an electron if you could actually *see* one. Remember, you can't look at an electron really because, like a wave, it is always moving and you stand no chance of predicting where an electron will be. Why not? This is because it will move by the time you figure out its location. This concept is called the **Heisenberg Uncertainty Principle.**

<u>The Heisenberg Uncertainty Principle is this</u>: you cannot possibly know the position of an electron and its energy state or momentum. It would look like this:

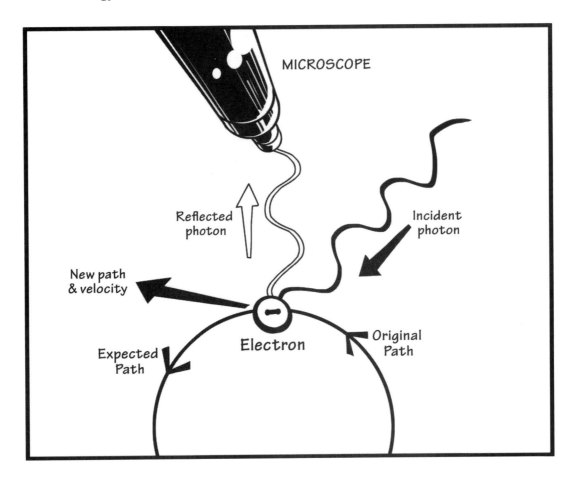

See how the act of *looking* messes up the path and velocity of an electron? This is why you can't expect a circular or predictable path—only a space (called an orbital) where an electron probably will be. Get it?

Electrons also have a *spin* to them. It isn't like a spinning top. The spin can only go two ways: *spin-up* (positive spin) and *spin-down* (negative spin). The thing to remember here is that <u>each orbital around a nucleus can have only two electrons</u>. Not only that, this is what at atom likes best: two electrons only per orbital, but one with a <u>positive spin</u> and one with a <u>negative spin</u>. This balanced state is low energy and preferable to the atom.

Electron Configuration and Arrangement

What does an orbital look like if not a circle as in the planetary orbits? Actually, it depends on the orbital. There are different orbital shapes that get much more complicated the larger an atom gets. If there are just a couple of electrons to deal with, there only needs to be one orbital (with room for two electrons only). This is the case for hydrogen and helium (which have one and two electrons only, respectively). Let's see what they look like:

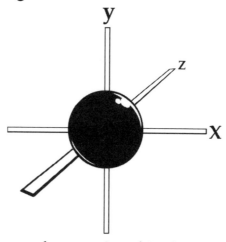

Hydrogen or Helium 1s Orbital

1s atomic orbital

So, it's basically a sphere in which one or two electrons can live. Hydrogen has one electron in this orbital (called the 1s) orbital; helium has two electrons in the same orbital. Remember that atoms are much happier with filled orbitals (two electrons per orbital)? They are happy with two matching electrons that they stick to themselves and don't interact with other atoms. Why is this important?

It's important because it determines if an atom/element will react or interact with others. Hydrogen atoms hate having one electron by itself _so much_ that they automatically react with other atoms. The idea is to have each atom use its single electron to pair with another atom (that also has a spare electron). See in this image how they are sharing in a hydrogen gas molecule so that each atom is happier (has a lower energy state, actually) with a neighbor than it is by itself:

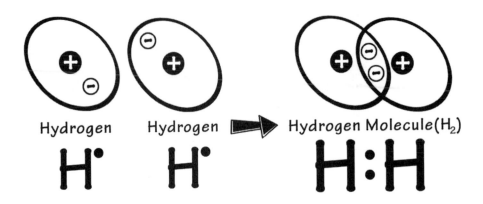

Hydrogen   Hydrogen ➡ Hydrogen Molecule(H₂)

H·   H·   H:H

Helium is different. It has two electrons (one with a positive spin and one with a negative spin) in the 1s orbital. This is a comfortable low-energy state already. Helium atoms have no room for other electrons, so they don't bother sharing. _This is why you will never see helium pairing with any other molecule for any natural reason._ Helium is one of the noble gases which naturally have filled orbitals and no desire to share them. This is what it looks like with its 1s orbital:

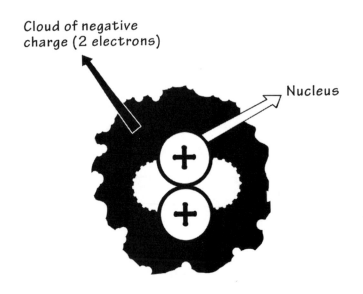

Cloud of negative charge (2 electrons)

Nucleus

Helium Atom

What if you have more than two electrons to deal with? All bigger elements must deal with this issue. There are many orbitals possible. These are bigger than the 1s orbital and extend outward from the nucleus. You will call them the 2s and 3s orbitals. There are nodes involved which are spaces we know have no chance of having any electrons.

They look like this:

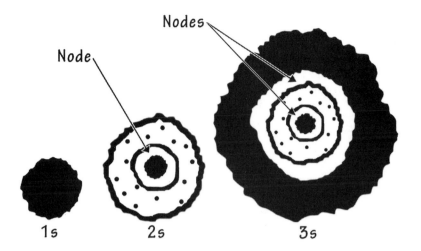

This Saturn-ring-like system looks great, but it doesn't work well to do this indefinitely. Why not? Because having so many electrons far away from the nucleus isn't exactly a low-energy state. Opposites attract in atoms, too; a negatively-charged electron is most stable as close to the proton as it can get. This problem is solved by having other orbital shapes that allow the electrons to live more happily in the lowest energy state possible.

This is what these strange-looking orbitals look like:

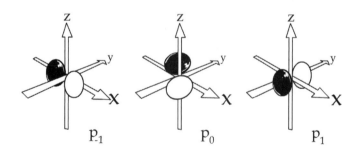

These are the p orbitals. They too like to have two electrons in each orbital. It starts to look a lot like an odd hotel with rooms called orbitals. In each orbital is a bunk bed with space for one electron on each bunk of these beds (two per bed).There are three sets of these p orbitals for each of the 3D axes (x, y, and z axes).

It gets crazier because with s orbitals and p orbitals only, you have enough room for a few more electrons. This means that atoms must get creative and have orbitals that need to be more oddly-shaped in order to have enough space for all of the electrons. Keep in mind here that the mathematical decision-making for electron probability is based on maintaining the lowest resting energy states possible. Two other orbital shapes are the d orbitals and f orbitals:

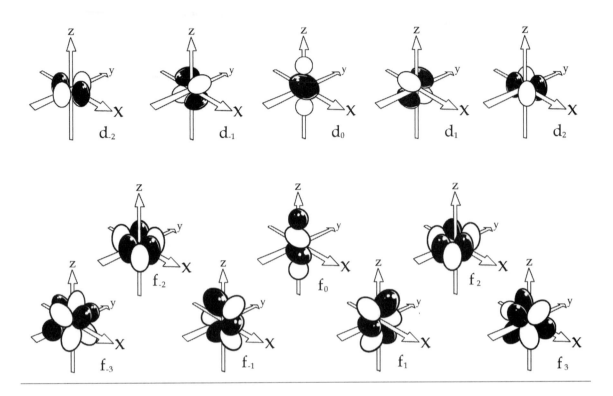

So, this odd arrangement of atomic hotel rooms just keeps getting filled up one-by-one as the elements get bigger and bigger. When we talk about the probability of an electron being in one place or another, you need to remember three things:

1. Each orbital must have no more than two electrons each.
2. Electrons must live in an orbital (they cannot just go about randomly).
3. The lowest energy state is preferred at all times.

The final piece that seals the deal for how atoms look and where electrons actually live inside them is not as orderly as you'd think. Atoms will always start with the 1s orbital and then the 2s orbital, filling electrons as the atoms get bigger. Then, however, the 3s orbital is not as energetically favorable as the three p orbitals. They get filled first, and then the 3s orbital gets its turn. You can see how this proceeds in an orderly (but not in the way you'd think) sort of way—allowing for atoms of very large elements to take up residence around the nucleus in these orbitals (that do not resemble planetary orbits at all).

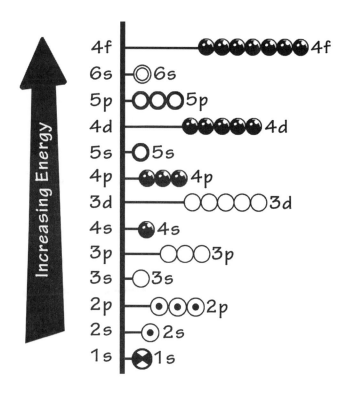

So, you need to use your imagination to see atoms as they really are (according to quantum mechanics and mathematical probability formulas). They are complex (but really beautiful, in an odd sort of chemistry way).

Atomic Mass and Related Terms

The atomic mass of any element is important to know. You have already learned how to use it in calculations, so we will touch on how it works and why it isn't the round number you'd expect at the lab bench. The atomic mass is the mass of an atom in units called ***atomic mass units*** (*abbreviated amu or u*).

There are a few terms related to atomic mass that seem similar but are actually different chemical terms you should know:

- **Atomic mass**—the mass of one atom of any element (so small you can't use anything but Daltons or atomic mass units to describe it); Daltons and atomic mass units are the same things.

- **Atomic number**—the number of protons in an element or atom. You use this number to see where an element is on the periodic table.

- **Mass number**—the number of protons and neutrons in an atom. It is also called the baryon number and will depend on what isotope you are talking about. For example, Carbon-12 is the commonest carbon type. It has 6 neutrons and 6 protons and a mass number of 12. Carbon-14 (with two extra neutrons) has a mass number of 14.

- **Molecular mass**—the same as the atomic mass unit but is the mass of any molecule made of any number of atoms.

- **Isotope mass (or isotopic mass)**— the mass of any isotope of an atom. It should be in atomic mass units and will be unique to the isotope.

- **Molar mass**—the mass of an average mole of any element or molecular substance (in grams per mole).

- **Average atomic mass**—the number you use to calculate how much of something is in a mole. It is averaged out and considers that any element in nature will have a certain percentage of different isotopes in it. Carbon's average mass is 12.0107 u (Daltons) and not an even 12 as you'd expect (from 6 neutrons and 6 protons). This is because there are isotopes in nature that, on average, offset this perfectly round number.

> *Let's discuss this:* For all practical purposes, the average atomic mass of an element and its molar mass are the same numbers. The average mass is in Daltons and the molar mass is in grams per mole, but Avogadro's number is factored in to make these two different number scales the same.

Let's Wrap This Up

Atoms are more complicated than you probably thought, but isn't everything when you take a closer look at it? The study of orbitals might not make sense to you now, but as you look at how chemical bonds are made and how the periodic table works, you'll see how it all comes together to make a great deal more sense.

In the next chapter, a whole lot more will be clearer as you learn the periodic table and study further how what you've learned so far fits into how this table works. As a budding chemist, you should see how the periodic table is really handy in opening up the world of chemistry with just one glance.

CHAPTER 4:

THE PERIODIC TABLE

This is the chapter you've been waiting for—the part where you get to know the different elements personally and understand exactly why they are in this table in the order they are. It's really amazing that nature figured out a way to make elements that were so orderly that they could be numbers from 1 to 118 in ways that will make a lot more sense very soon.

Periodic Table Properties and Trends

Finally, we get to the periodic table in this chapter. This table is the key to understanding most things you need to know about chemistry. It contains every known element in specific rows (called periods) and columns (called groups), starting one-by-one with the smallest element first and the largest element last. This means that the atomic mass goes up by one as you read each element in turn.

Outside of rare and mostly transient gigantic atoms at the bottom of the table (which get discovered once in a while), we know that there are no missed elements. If there were, there would be a missing box on the periodic table. As it is, every box is accounted for.

Not all of the elements had been discovered when a Russian chemist named Dmitri Mendeleev in the late 1860s decided to order the known elements. When he figured out the key to doing this, he realized that they were arranged in an extremely unique way. When he started putting the collection of elements into the table, he was able to see where there were spaces that existed between the known elements. These were filled in over the past 150 years or so as more elements were discovered.

To be clear, Mendeleev did not invent the periodic table: he just uncovered what was already there. What he came up with and what you will soon learn yourself was a clever way of ordering the elements that makes the greatest possible sense. This is how it works:

- The periodic table is _ordered by the atomic number_ (from 1 to 118). The atomic number is the number of protons in an atom of the element. Because atoms are generally electrically neutral, this is also the number of electrons in each atom.

- _Each element is given an atomic symbol._ Some are easy to remember, such as H for hydrogen or C for carbon. Others are much harder, like Ag for silver or K for potassium. These should be memorized for the most common elements.

- _The atomic mass is on the table near the atomic symbol._ Remember that the atomic mass is in Daltons or amu. It won't be an even integer because of isotopes that affect the average atomic mass of a large sample of atoms (and every sample you'd use in the lab would be considered large by atomic standards). Only the average neutron count affects this number, as the atomic number (number of protons) needs to stay the same for each atom of the same element. This is what you'll see in each square:

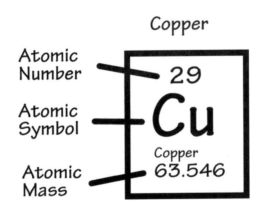

Let's look at the table itself. It is arranged with 7 rows or periods and 18 Groups (columns). In order to condense its shape a bit, some of the elements have been extracted out of the middle and are instead displayed at the bottom. If this wasn't done, the table would make far less sense.

Understanding the Rows or Periods

Why is the periodic table shaped the way it is? Actually, it all comes back to the orbitals around each atomic neutron. Isolating the first three periods will help you see why this works the way it does:

First Three Periods =
First Three Atomic Orbital Levels

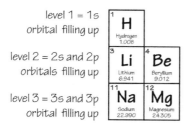

Remember that the 1s orbital is all you'll need for hydrogen and helium (the first period/level). Two electrons fill this orbital. Hydrogen has just one of these, and helium has 2, which fill up that level. The next two levels have both s orbitals and p orbitals on the outer *shell*, so to speak. There are inner-shell electrons on the 1s orbital, but the ones that interact with other atoms are the outer-shell or *upper-level* electrons. There is room for 6 electrons in the p orbitals (remember, there are three of these per energy level) and 2 electrons in the 2s orbital at that level. That makes eight spots, which is exactly how many elements are in each row (levels 2 and 3).

It isn't until you get to the next level that the d orbitals are needed. How does that look, and does it fit with what we know about the d orbitals (that aren't needed until the 4th period)?

Periods 4 and 5 of the Periodc Table

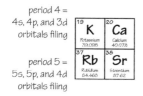

There are a total of 5 d orbitals per level/period. That makes 10 spots for electrons. Add the 6 spots in the p orbitals and the 2 spots in the s orbitals. This adds to a total of 18 spots for electrons. This is precisely the number of groups or spaces you'll see in these two rows.

- 5s - 1 orbital

- 5p - 3 orbitals

- 5d - 5 orbitals

Of course, after that are the rows with f orbitals, which have room for a total of 14 electrons. This is where you get the lanthanides and actinides (explained below), which would add 14 squares to the 6th and 7th periods. You can see why these 14 squares are accounted for (because of the 7 f orbitals making up 14 spaces for electrons):

Lanthanides and Actinides at Bottom of Table
(but fit inside periods 6 and 7)

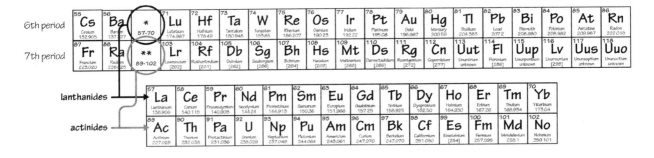

So, the table is precisely what it should look like, row-by-row. The elements are arranged by electron-energy levels, with each element down the row adding one more electron. As you get to the end of the row, you come to the noble gases (like helium, xenon, and neon). These have totally filled energy levels, so they do not tend to react much at all with anything. They have no room or desire to have electrons added or removed from their outer shells.

Understanding the Columns or Groups

Now, how about the columns, or *groups*?

The groups are actually more interesting and tell you more about what kind of element you are dealing with. Broadly classified, there are three groups you must learn about in the periodic table. These are the _metals, metalloids,_ and _nonmetals_. They don't line up nicely in the periodic table but form jagged lines that cross the table like this:

Metal elements conduct electricity, while nonmetals do not. Metalloids have confusing properties of both metals and nonmetals. These properties can be found in the different substances:

- _Metals_—solid, shiny, conduct metal, malleable, conduct electricity, and likely to lose electrons readily (this is important in why they like to form ions and make salts).
- _Metalloids_—also called _semimetals_; these are semiconductors, have may different forms, and may lose or gain electrons in forming bonds.
- _Nonmetals_—brittle and non-conductive of electricity; likely to gain electrons in bonding and reactions; have lower melting points than metallic elements.

Within each category, there are many subcategories that have similar characteristics. In general, the elements in the same group are much more alike than any elements in the same period. You will see why this is the case in short order.

Let's first look at the different types of substances in the periodic table:

Periodic Table of the Elements

- **Alkali metals.** These are lithium, sodium, potassium, rubidium, cesium, and francium (group 1A on the table or the first column). As pure metals, they are very soft and react strongly with water (remember what happens with sodium metal and water?). Most of these metals exist in nature as salts (ions) because they readily bind to nonmetals, like chloride or bromide. Even though hydrogen is in group 1A, it isn't a metal at all.

- **Alkaline-earth metals.** The alkaline-earth metals are mainly Group 2 in the periodic table. Commonly-known metals of this class are beryllium, magnesium, calcium, strontium, barium, and radium. There are two extra electrons in the outer shell (as you would know because they are in the second spot from the left). This means they are less reactive than group 1A metals while still being reactive. These often form metal ions in salts, similar to the alkali metals.

- **Lanthanides.** This group is messier and isn't on the table as the other groups are laid out. This is the group with elements 57 through 70. Look for them at the bottom of the table above the actinides. You will rarely encounter any of these elements in a laboratory or even in nature. There are 14 lanthanides in the sixth period of the table.

- **Actinides.** The actinides are below the lanthanides on the periodic table and represent elements numbers 89 to 103. You'll find thorium and uranium on this row, which occur naturally in amounts you can mine (these are radioactive). Together with the lanthanides, this collection is called the *inner transition metal group.*

Things to know: If an element can't be found in nature or doesn't last longer than a fraction of a second, does it really count? This is an interesting question. Some of the heavier elements above atomic number 100 were created in a lab in order to "discover" them. Once discovered, the chemists had to look fast to see them as they lasted only a brief period of time before disintegrating due to their radioactivity. Oh, and they got to name their very own element. These are interesting but impractical in the study of chemistry.

- **Transition metals.** This is a swath of metals in the middle of the table; they include 38 different metals. Among the common ones are titanium, manganese, iron, cobalt, nickel, copper, zinc, silver, cadmium, gold, tungsten, platinum, and mercury. These are the metals you most think of as being *metallic.*

- **Post transition metals.** These are things like tin, lead, bismuth, and aluminum (extending from groups 13 through 17 of the periodic table). They are softer and do not conduct metal as well as the transition metals.

- **Metalloids.** These are in-between elements, including arsenic, silicon, boron, antimony, and polonium. These are elements drifting toward the nonmetals on the righthand side of the periodic table. Some are used in industry as semiconductors (especially boron and silicon).

- **Nonmetals.** This is the group near the right side of the periodic table. Nonmetals include carbon, phosphorus, nitrogen, sulfur, oxygen, and selenium. Even hydrogen in group 1 is a nonmetal (but for different reasons).

- **Halogens.** Halogens are a subset of nonmetals. These are important in making many salts you see in nature. Common halogens are fluorine, chlorine, bromine, and iodine.

These are very chemically reactive (just like the alkali metals they often combine with to make salts). Look for many examples of pairing up alkali metals and halogens in nature.

- **Noble gases.** These are *noble* because they exist by themselves and rarely interact with other substances. They are mainly inert gases in group 18 and include xenon, neon, argon, and helium. Element 119 hasn't been *discovered* yet but if so, it would be a very short-lived gaseous substance.

Making Sense of Periodic Table Trends

The beauty of the periodic table is best appreciated when you see the different trends within the table itself. After you master these trends, you will feel like you are really well on your way to becoming more than a junior chemist. These are the trends to keep track of:

- **Ionic Radius Trend**: The ionic radius is the relative size of the atom if it becomes ionized (turns into a charged ion). This is appreciated by the table shown below. The ionic radius shrinks because of two factors. The first is having a small size. If an atom is small, its ionic radius will be small. The second is the number of electrons in the outer shell. If the outer shell has a lot of electrons, its ionic radius will shrink, and it will not give up these electrons readily. The ionic radius will be a little bigger or a little smaller than the radius of the atom in its neutral state.

  On the lefthand side, you'll see cations (positively charged ions) because, as you'll remember, these charged molecules have extra electrons, but just a few of them. They are more likely to give these away than they are to collect them. Why? Because it's easier to give away one or two electrons (and be positively charged) than it is to add 6 or 7 of them (to fill all 8 orbital slots in the first few rows).

  Anions are on the right. They have 6 or 7 electrons out of the 8 electrons they need to fill the complete number of desired electron spots (octet) in the outer shell. It is better/easier for these to become anions by stealing a couple of electrons than it would be to get rid of those extra ones they have.

Periodic Trends

recall: trends

Periodic Table & Trends

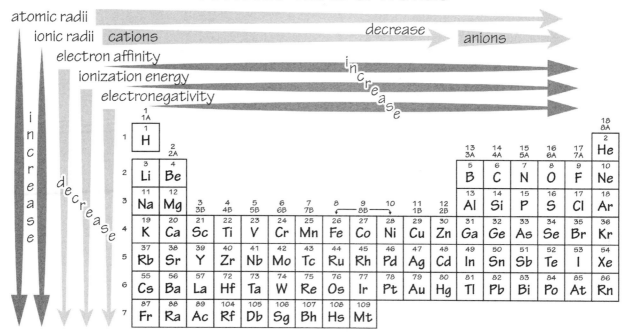

- **Ionization energy trend.** This also a trend you'll want to follow. The ionizing energy is the amount of energy an atom must absorb to let go of an electron. The first electron on the outer shell is easier to discharge than the second or third electrons. This is a stepwise increase in energy as more electrons are released. It explains why it is too hard to ionize more than a few electrons together and why most cations are charged just +1 or +2. The ionization energy follows the same trend as electron affinity. The greater the electron affinity an atom has, the higher is its ionization energy. It means the highest electron affinity and greatest ionization energy occur in the upper righthand corner of the periodic table.

- **Electronegativity trend.** This is a trend that increases from the lower left to the upper righthand side of the table. This is a measure of how attractive the atom is to any electrons available to it from other atoms. A highly electronegative element like fluorine is small, dense, and missing a full *octet* of electrons in its outer shell. For this reason, it desires to attract electrons and vice versa greatly. It forms a negatively charged ion (F-) easily and is reactive with positively charged metals, like Na+ (sodium ion). If there is a large electronegativity difference between atoms, they will form ions and won't truly *share* electrons. They form what are called ionic bonds. Those with similar electronegativity values will form covalent bonds, which involve greater levels of sharing between atoms.

- **Atomic radius trend.** The atomic radius is hard to measure. It is sometimes described as the closest distance you can get to an atom without bonding to it. This is known as the van der Waals radius. There are other options, such as the metallic radius—between two identical metals in a crystal lattice. In addition, the ionic radius is one-half the distance between two dissimilar ions that are just touching. This increases in a downward and rightward trend.

So this is the periodic table in a nutshell. Now that you see how it comes together and the trends within it, a great deal more about how bonds are made and why will be crystal clear.

Isotopes of Elements

The elements on the periodic table are ordered by atomic number (proton number). While you can't add protons to an element and keep the same element name, you can add or take away neutrons without affecting much. Neutrons weigh roughly the same as protons but they are neutral in charge, so they don't affect the element's electrical neutrality. When the neutron count is changed, the weight of the atom is altered as well. These altered-weight atoms are isotopes.

All elements have some isotopes. Hydrogen, for example, has two isotopes, called deuterium and tritium. They look like this:

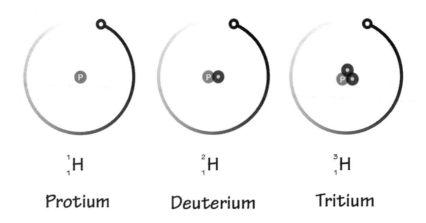

$^{1}_{1}\text{H}$ $^{2}_{1}\text{H}$ $^{3}_{1}\text{H}$

Protium   Deuterium   Tritium

Note the differences in the atomic nucleus and the change in weight of the atom (but not its charge).

Isotopes were first discovered in the early 1900s when researchers began to study radioactivity. Radioactive decay involves changing one element into another by changing its nucleus. Tritium does this and *miraculously* becomes helium by adding an electron and changing a neutron into a proton. It looks like this:

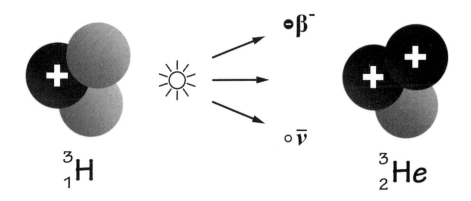

Fun Science: Tritium gives off an electron which is a wave you can't see in the visible spectrum. If you put tritium into a vial and coat the inside of the vial with phosphor, the phosphor will glow in the visible spectrum so you can see it. While this means it is radioactive, it is perfectly safe. You might see it in real life as it causes fancy watches and exit signs to glow.

Radioactivity and radioactive substances are not the same as isotopes. This is because radioactive processes involve the actual *switching* of elements rather than changing the size of a nucleus by adding a neutron. Again, adding a proton changes the element, but adding a neutron keeps the element with the same name (but different weight).

Other researchers looked at neon gas and found that it gave off different positive ray beams. This meant the gas must be made from atoms of various sizes. The research ultimately culminated in finding neon-20 and neon-22 in 1919. The two numbers refer to the atomic mass of the neon atoms.

Given the atomic number of 10 for neon, you can see where neon-20 has 10 neutrons, and neon-22 has 11 neutrons. Because the listed mass for this element on the periodic table is 20.180, you know that most of the atoms in any random sample of neon gas are neon-20. Remember the atomic mass is a weighted average. The number you see is closer to 20 than it is to 22.

Most isotopes are stable and not likely to randomly lose or gain any neutrons. In extreme circumstances, like in a nuclear reactor or inside stars, however, isotopes may get the energy they need to become unstable. Strange things like fusion and fission/splitting of atoms occur.

What happens, for example, inside stars like our sun? These are gigantic masses that are under a great deal of gravitational pressure. Deep inside them, the temperature and pressure are so huge that the hydrogen inside these stars actually fuses to make helium gas (plus energy). This is the same energy given off by *hydrogen bombs*. The difference is that stars do this over time and don't explode in the same way. This chemical/atomic fusion process looks like this:

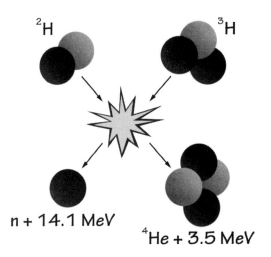

^{2}H ^{3}H

n + 14.1 MeV

^{4}He + 3.5 MeV

Real-World Applications: *Carbon-14 is a naturally occurring radioactive isotope of carbon. It is found in everything but only 1 part in a trillion of all carbon atoms. It has a known half-life of 5,730 years, meaning half is gone after that period of time. When it decays, it becomes nitrogen-14 plus energy. By measuring the amount of C-14 in an organic substance, you can see how old it is with reasonable accuracy.*

Making Molecules out of Elements

The next chapter will be about the bonding of elements. There is no such thing as a generic chemical bond. There are different types of bonds between atoms; it all depends on their chemistry. Most bonding you'll come across will involve the first few rows of the periodic table (mostly s and p orbitals).

When two atoms decide to pair, a couple of things control what the interaction looks like. One is the electronegativity of the atoms involved; the other is the types of orbitals involved. The orbitals we've talked about will not be the same after bonding. They will give rise to what are called *hybrid orbitals*. We will look at what these look like in a minute.

As you will learn, electrons are only shared equally if there are two atoms involved that are precisely the same. Hydrogen gas, for example, is easy because it involves two identical hydrogen atoms equally sharing a single electron. The bond they form involves two s orbitals; it's called a sigma bond. Sigma bonds look like this:

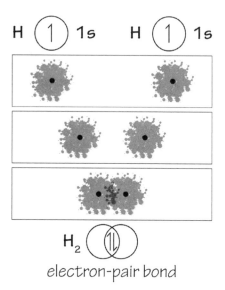

electron-pair bond

The sharing of electrons in this bond occurs only because <u>the energy state involved in the sharing is less than the energy that exists should each electron remain separate</u>. It's a matter of the distance between two positively charged nuclei being *just right*. If the distance is too great, the 1s orbitals can't even overlap. If it's too close, the charged nuclei will repel each other. If you look at an energy diagram with energy versus distance measured, you will get a lower energy (preferred) state at the distance these atoms exist as a diatomic molecule:

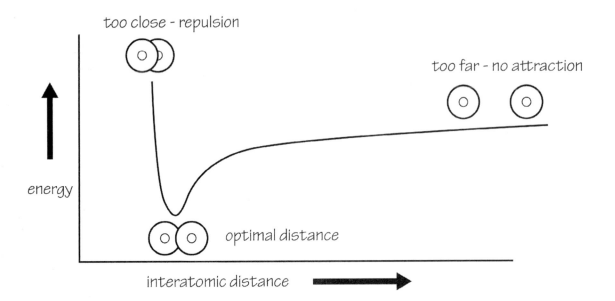

too close - repulsion

too far - no attraction

energy

optimal distance

interatomic distance

The lowest energy state in the diagram becomes the *bond length*. You can imagine the sigma bond as being shaped like two balloons squashed together. Very simply, it would look like this:

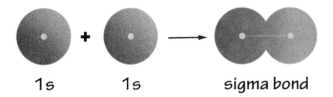

1s   1s   sigma bond

Sigma bonds can get more complex than this, however, especially when it comes to larger atoms and bonding between dissimilar atoms. Any two orbitals (s or p) that attach by touching the orbitals in an end-on way will become a sigma bond: an s and p orbital can make a sigma bond, or 2 p orbitals can make one (as long as they are end-on as they connect to one another) like these:

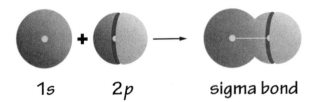

1s   2p   sigma bond

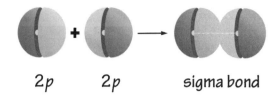

2p   2p   **sigma bond**

The situation with two p orbitals making a sigma bond is what it looks like when two fluorine atoms combine their half-filled 2p orbitals to make a sigma bond between them.

There are very complex orbital shapes in organic chemistry, where carbon and nitrogen bind with many other different molecules. These often involve s and p orbitals mixing together in complex ways. Take the case of carbon, for example. It has four electrons in its outer energy shell (at the second energy level). These four will fill out half of the available slots. The 2s orbital gets filled first, leaving 2 left for the remaining p orbitals like this:

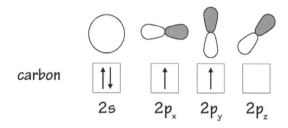

With the carbon nucleus in the middle, there are 4 electrons spaced out as far as possible from one another (because they repel each other, right?). This leads to a tetrahedral shape of any molecule with carbon in the middle. These orbitals mix together to make four bonding *hybrid* orbitals, called sp3 orbitals. They look like this:

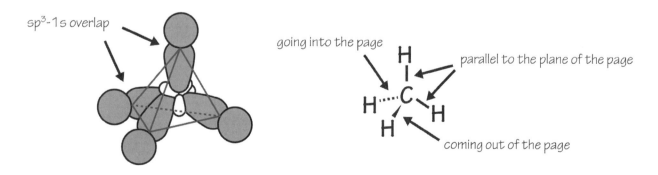

tetrahedral sp³ bonding in methane

Can you see the tetrahedral shape? These funky orbitals allow any atoms attached to the central carbon atom to be as far apart from one another as they can.

Nitrogen is another common atom in nature. It has 5 electrons in its outer shell. This stretches out, as you can see in the image. There is one lone pair by themselves plus three spread out over the p orbitals. This lone pair of electrons take up its own space, so the rest of the electrons are spread out in a pyramidal shape. The bonds between nitrogen and other atoms are in this shape:

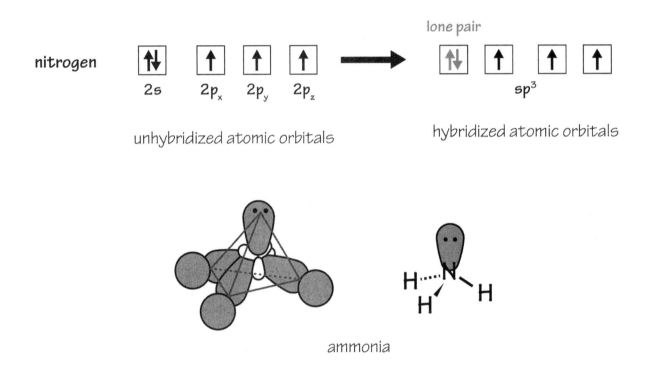

unhybridized atomic orbitals

hybridized atomic orbitals

ammonia

Let's do one more like this so you can see how complex it might be. Oxygen has 6 spare electrons in the same shell (called the valence shell). As the electrons spread out, you get the availability of 2 spare electrons that _will not_ bond to other atoms straight out to the side. This is because there are two lone pairs of electrons to account for. The shape is tetrahedral, but the bond is called _bent_:

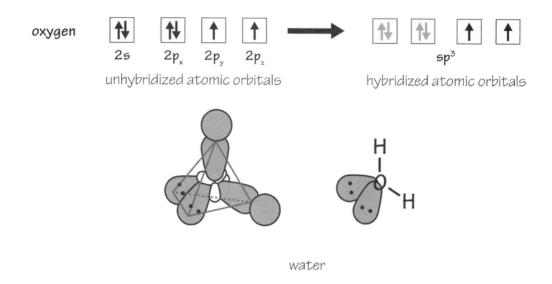

In the above example, you see how oxygen and hydrogen make water. You can now see exactly why the H2O water molecule is naturally bent.

Besides the sigma bonds and these hybrid orbitals, you can also get what are called pi bonds. They can happen with two p orbitals that cannot bind end-on-end. Instead, the p orbitals graze each other from the side. See what a pi bond looks like in a molecule of ethene, which has a sigma bond plus a pi bond to make two _double bonds_ between the carbon atoms:

The other feature that determines what a bond looks like is the electronegativity difference between two dissimilar atoms. Note that the bond depends on the _difference_ between each atom and not on a specific electronegativity value. A big difference means the bond will be ionic; a small difference means it will be covalent. We will talk a lot about these bonds next. For now, you need to know that ionic bonds are those where the electrons are not shared very equally, while covalent bonds have the sharing of electrons more evenly.

The electronegativity of an atom is a scored number. You can find tables of the electronegativity values for each element. The higher the number, the stronger the atom pulls at other electrons in order to grab them for bonding. If you take two atoms and find the difference between their electronegativity values, you can decide if the bond will be ionic, covalent, or in-between (called polar covalent bonding). This is what you should look for:

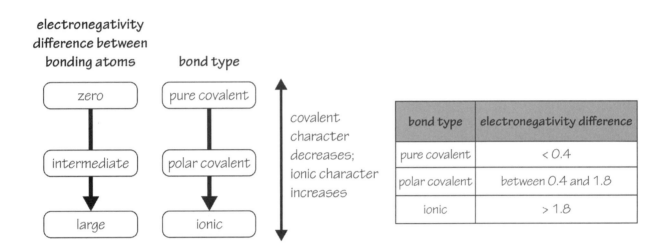

Let's Wrap This Up

The periodic table is a work of genius, even as no one actually invented it. It invented itself by the natural order of the 118 known elements. The more you understand the table, the better able you will be to see how atoms form molecules through bonding and why the inert noble elements have no desire to do this. Study the trends you see in the table; this will take you far in understanding the behavior of each element.

You will study more about the bonding between the elements next. From what you've learned so far, there are reasons why certain elements form specific bond types preferentially over other types. Now that you understand the table better, you should be more comfortable looking at two elements and seeing exactly which bonds they are likely to make.

SECTION 3:
CHEMICAL BONDS

Since so many atoms and elements are found in nature as molecules rather than atoms, you should take the time to learn about chemical bonds. There are big differences in bond strength and properties; these are related strongly to the physics of each atom type and the need for all atoms to exist in a low-energy state. Bonds are made to lower the energy of an atomic/molecular system.

Breaking chemical bonds is the basis for a great many chemical reactions. As you will see, some of these reactions will involve putting energy into the system (to break the bonds); others happen spontaneously because the energy in the new products of the chemical reaction is less than the energy in the starting substrates.

CHAPTER 5:

IONIC BONDING

Ionic bonds are common. These are the types of bonds that become salts once the bond has formed. Ionic bonding is best described as an unequal sharing of electrons between two atoms. One atom hogs one or more electrons from another atom, leaving two atoms that are both very happy with the outcome. Let's look at what ions are and how they form these crucial mismatched bonds.

Ions

While an atom of any element has the potential to be electrically neutral, this is not the state in which many prefer to be in the natural world. The different groups or columns of the periodic table provide clues to you about the state they most desire.

For example, take group 1A, which are the alkali metals (sodium, lithium, and potassium, mainly). These have circulating electrons with a single electron sitting by itself in the outer valence shell. This simplified drawing of sodium shows its single outer valence shell electron:

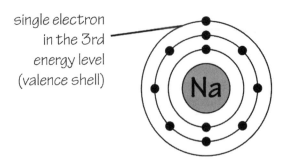

sodium as a neutral atom

single electron in the 3rd energy level (valence shell)

In this image, you have an electrically-neutral atom that is not happy this way. It would be in a far lower energy state if it could essentially eliminate the valence electron (and give it to another atom). The ion (written as Na+) is one where the electron is readily shared with another atom. It shares best with other atoms that want to accept an electron and one that would be in a lower energy state by taking sodium's extra electron.

Sodium is like all other group 1 atoms that are in the perfect position to lose the electron they have in their outer shell. All they need is another atom that wants to catch an electron as badly as these atoms want to get rid of it. One of the best answers to this problem is an atom belonging to group 17, which are the halogens.

Here is chlorine on the opposite side of the periodic table—a halogen. It has the opposite problem as sodium. With 7 of 8 desired electrons in its outer shell, it could easily use an electron to fill its valence shell. The atom would be in a more optimal energy state with an electron:

chlorine as a neutral atom

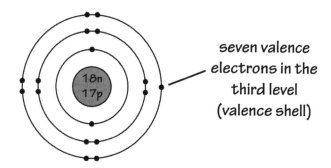

seven valence electrons in the third level (valence shell)

When these two molecules get together, their sharing is beneficial for each other. In a simplified form, it looks like this:

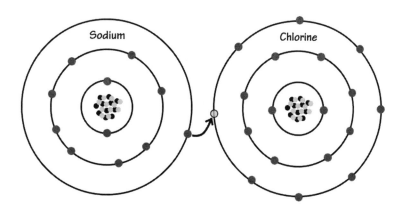

The end result is the molecule we know as sodium chloride or *table salt*.

As you can see, an ion can be positively charged or negatively charged. An anion is any negatively-charged atom, while a cation is any positively-charged atom. Being a matched pair of positive and negative substances, these will attract one another like all electrically-charged things. All anions have an excess of electrons versus protons, while all cations have a deficiency of electrons versus protons. You know an atom is an ion by the plus sign (+ for cations) or minus sign (- for anions) after the symbol.

You should recognize too that the group 2 atoms (column 2 of the periodic table) are also very likely to ionize with 2 electrons in the outer valence shell. These elements are the ones that form 2+ cations when they give up these two electrons to another atom or group of atoms that want to take them. You end up with salts such as $CaCl_2$ which involves one Ca^{2+} cation and 2 Cl^- anions.

Outside of these two groups, you will also get odd combinations of cations, such as NH_4^+ (ammonium ion), NO_2^+ (nitronium), and even H_3O^+ (hydronium ion). Look for these ions functioning in ways similar to the traditional single-atom ions.

Some metals are unique and able to form more than one type of cation. These often do not have a +/- symbol after them but instead have Roman numerals, such as I, II, and III. Iron (II) is called the ferrous ion, while iron (III) is called the ferric ion. The suffix (-ous) is often for the ion with the lower number of valence electrons around it, while the suffix (-ic) is often for the ion with the higher number of valence electrons around it. Copper, tin, iron, manganese, lead, and chromium all have this feature. These are more complex to explain as there are more than just s and p orbitals involved.

Nitrates and nitrites, as well as sulfates and sulfites, are examples of different but similar anions. Nitrite, for example, is NO_2^-, and nitrate is NO_3^-. In this case, the suffix *-ite* is used for the anion with less oxygen, and the suffix *-ate* is used for the anion with more oxygen involved in these *oxyanion* compounds.

There is a special situation called a *zwitterion* which is seen in larger molecules like amino acids. A zwitterion is electrically neutral but has a positive charge somewhere in it and a negative charge elsewhere in the same molecule. You can sometimes think of a zwitterion as a molecule with an electron flitting back and forth between two spots on the molecule. A zwitterion looks like this:

An ion is made by the process of *ionization,* which essentially means gain or losing electrons. It is not possible in nature to have an electron randomly given away without some other substance (an atom, in this case) accepting it. This is how it works in chemical systems on a molecular basis, when atoms become ionized, sharing their electrons with other atomic substances.

Ions do not have to be single atoms; they can be polyatomic, where a small group of atoms as a group together become a functional ion. These include things like $SO_4{}^{2-}$ or the *sulfate anion.* Together, these five atoms look like this:

sulfate ion

Anions are negatively-charged ions. Common anions are the halogens like F-, Cl-, Br-, and I-. There are many others. Oxide is O^{2-}, hydride is H-, and nitride is N^{2-}. Oxygen is particularly active in making polyatomic anions, such as phosphate ($PO_4{}^{2-}$), nitrite ($NO_2{}^-$), and sulfite ($SO_3{}^{2-}$). The list of these is long, largely because oxygen is so reactive with multiple other atoms.

Other odd ions are those starting with *hypo-* or *per-*. These are also oxyanions involving chlorine and oxygen. There are actually four of these:

- Hypochlorite = ClO-
- Chlorite = ClO2-
- Chlorate = ClO3-
- Perchlorate = ClO4-

These can get very complicated. Just so you can see how this turns out, these are the different chlorine-based oxyanions:

Hypochlorite   Chlorite   Chlorate   Perchlorate

Finally, there are hydrogen-based polyanions using bi- and di- as prefixes. These are things like bicarbonate (HCO3-) and bisulfate (HSO4-). You should try to memorize these as they are hard to determine otherwise.

You write salt formulas with the cation first and the anion second. In general, the cation is named as its regular atomic name, using words like sodium, lithium, and magnesium to call the first word of a two-word salt. The anion is second and isn't named in the same way. Many have the suffix of (-ide). This means that bromine becomes *bromide*, fluorine becomes *fluoride*, and oxygen becomes *oxide*. Others like sulfate or phosphate are named without changing the verbiage. It would look like this:

- Calcium plus oxygen = calcium oxide or CaO
- Ammonia (NH3) plus sulfate = ammonium sulfate or (NH4)2SO4 or $(NH_4)_2SO_4$
- Iron (II) plus oxygen = Fe(II)O or ferrous oxide
- Strontium plus chlorine = strontium chloride or SrCl2

In figuring out these salts, find the least electronegative ion (which is the cation) and the most electronegative ion (which is the anion). Figure out the desired charge for each, and balance the salt's name and symbol so the resulting salt will be completely electrically neutral.

Now that you know how salts are put together and why it is energetically favorable for certain atoms to make these kinds of mixed ionic molecules, let's look at the ionic bond itself.

Ionic Bond and Ionic Compounds

Ionic bonding can be thought of as a relatively complete transfer of one or more valence electrons between two atoms. It requires an electronegativity difference between two atoms great enough that one wishes to give up the ion, while the other wishes to take it. In many cases, the donor is a metallic element and the acceptor is a nonmetal. The charge you see on the ion directly reflects the number of electrons available for donation or acceptance. Once the ionic bond is formed, the overall salt will be electrically neutral.

For the first few rows of the periodic table, it's the *octet* you need to think about. This octet comes from a single s orbital and 3 p orbitals on each energy level. This adds up to enough room for 8 electrons; the lowest energy state comes from having the entire energy level filled up (however it does that). You can draw a dot structure (called a Lewis dot structure) that looks like this with sodium chloride:

In some cases, a single atom, such as magnesium (with 2 electrons to give up), will give one electron to one atom (like chlorine) and another to yet another atom (usually another chlorine). It will look like this:

Let's Wrap This Up

Ions and ionic bonding are common in chemistry. We will talk more about how ions dissolve in aqueous solutions, but you can see that with all of this free swapping of electrons, some of this exchange happens with the water molecule (the solvent) itself. This is exactly why aqueous solutions of ions conduct electricity. The conduction of electricity is nothing more than the travel of electrons from one place to another. Ions help this process by being so free in providing these electrons.

You should take away from this chapter how to identify ions, which ions are more likely to form molecules with other ions, and why this happens. Understand which atoms will bond ionically with which others and why. Learn how to name an ionic compound correctly. Practice putting together some ionic compounds and balancing them. Let's move on to other bonding types.

CHAPTER 6:

COVALENT BONDING

You can think of covalent bonding as two atoms playing together more nicely than in ionic bonding. There is increased sharing of the electrons each atom contributes to the mix. As you will see, there is a lot of leeway in what is called *covalent* versus what is called *ionic*. When in doubt about the type of bond to expect between two atoms, find their electronegativity values, subtract the values, and refer to the table in chapter 5 to see what type of bond is most likely present.

Covalent Bond

Covalent bonds are any bonds between two atoms where there is relative sharing of the electron pairs. This shared electron pair is called a *shared pair* or a *bonding pair*. As mentioned earlier, true and complete sharing of these electrons can only happen when the atoms between them are identical. We have talked about some of these bonds already, such as the sigma bond and pi bond.

In a double bond, such as between two carbon atoms, you will need one sigma and one pi bond. This is because there will only be one S orbital in the valence shell; the other orbital must be a P orbital. Again, with pi bonds, the p orbitals are not overlapping end-to-end but merely graze each other as they sit side-by-side.

All covalent bonds with dissimilar atoms must have some degree of polarity. What does polarity mean? Polarity means that one atom is pulling harder at the electron than the other.

This figure shows how we draw polarity in a polar covalent bond:

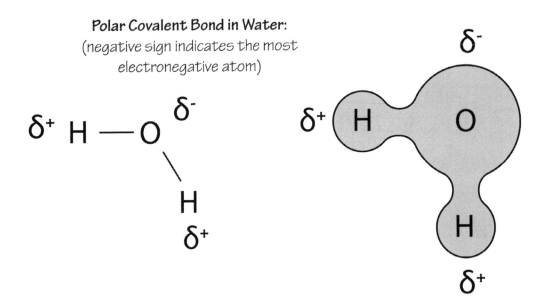

Polar Covalent Bond in Water:
(negative sign indicates the most electronegative atom)

A couple of things you need to know are that a single bond or sigma bond is the stronger of the two bonds, and, in a triple bond, you will see one sigma and two pi bonds. Pi bonds can be made with p orbitals as well as with d orbitals, neither of which make very strong bonds.

While ionic bonds form smaller molecules, covalent bonds can be a part of very large molecules, including macromolecules you see in biochemical structures. You will also see covalent bonding in certain gases, such as sulfur dioxide, carbon dioxide, and methane. These small, covalently-bonded structures have such a low boiling temperature that many are gaseous at room temperature. Others, like ethanol, are liquid at room temperature but have low boiling points. Giant structures, like starch and proteins, can be solid at room temperature and may not dissolve in water.

Is it possible to have more than one electron in these types of relationships? Absolutely! Take the case of nitric oxide, for example. This is made from nitrogen and oxygen, having a double bond between them. They actually have three electrons in this bond. This image shows you what it looks like:

See the top? There are 3 electrons that share this covalent bond. The gas we call oxygen or dioxygen can look a lot like this:

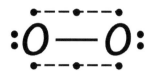

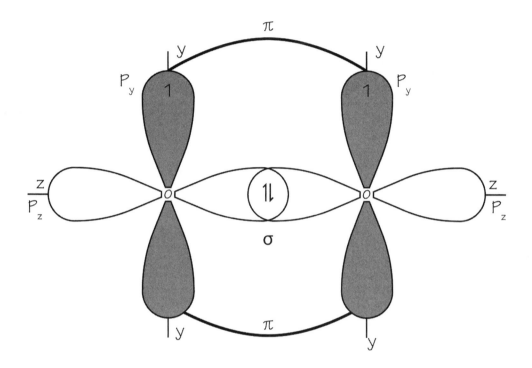

formation of π bond in O_2 molecule

You can see by this drawing how it might appear if you can look at the orbitals themselves. As you can see, there is one sigma bond and one pi bond. You need to understand that these molecules are often very reactive; however, because their electronegativities are similar, the bond between them is very stable.

Let's move on to resonance. This is seen in some molecules that have a single bond and a double bond coming off the same atom. Try to avoid thinking of these bonds as being extremely stable; instead, an electron might flit back and forth between a single bond and a double bond, so you couldn't tell which bond was double and which was single. This image shows you how it looks with NO3 or nitrate:

This looks messy; however, you need to think of the electron as being equally attracted to any of the three oxygen molecules in this structure.

Some organic molecules take resonance to a whole new level. These are often carbon-based circular/planar molecules that must satisfy what is called Huckel's rule, which states that there must be 4n +2 atoms in the ring where n is any integer, to create resonance. Most of the time, n = 1, so these will be resonant 6-membered rings. These molecules are called aromatic compounds. You will see aromaticity in things like benzene or phenol. This is what an aromatic structure looks like:

Benzene Aromatic Ring

Polarity

Polarity is interesting. As you can see by the water molecule earlier, the polar bond can be thought of as having the electron's charge between the atoms split and partially carried on either side of the bond. The charge created has a strength (size) plus a direction. This directional arrow/charge is called a dipole moment. You need to realize that, to remain polar, the molecule (such as water) must be of a certain geometry, _or the two opposite dipole moments will cancel each other out_. It wouldn't be polar anymore.

The dipole moment is not too difficult to understand. Take a molecule of water (H_2O), for example. IF the charge is split between the atoms and IF the molecule is lopsided itself (because of its geometry), there will be a tiny magnetic charge difference (the dipole moment) you can measure. Any molecule considered polar has this magnetic charge. It's what allows molecules like water to help conduct electricity AND to attract other polar molecules using other bonding (to be discussed next). The dipole moment for water is shown here:

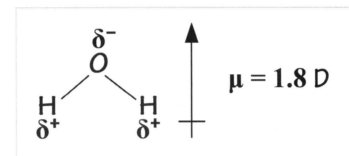

The dipole moment depends on the charge differences in the molecule AND the distance between the charges. The higher the charge and the larger the difference, the higher this number is. The symbol you see (delta δ) means "partial charge," while the symbol mu (μ) is the size or magnitude of the total charge on the molecule. The unit of measure is the Debye unit, which is an extremely small amount of magnetism. ***NOTE: The arrow will point to the more electronegative end of the molecule.***

An element with a high degree of electronegativity is said to be very *electron greedy*. Imagine this atom matching with an atom that isn't so greedy. This is what you see with things like oxygen, chlorine, and fluorine (with high electronegativities). If they mix with atoms like the alkali metals or alkaline earth metals (with very low electronegativities), you'll have a situation where one atom wants the electron and the other is more than willing to give it away. Again, at one extreme, the bond will be ionic (electronegativity difference of greater than 2.0); at the other extreme, the bond will be covalent and nonpolar (Electronegativity difference of less than 0.5 between atoms).

Remember this: Polarity is not the same thing as electronegativity. You will call a molecule "polar" if there is a dipole moment or a net charge on the molecule itself. Any molecule (like CO_2) will have differences in electronegativity between atoms, but it won't be polar. This is because, as mentioned, there isn't a dipole moment (they cancel each other out).

So, when you want to know if a molecule is polar or nonpolar, you need to know not only the electronegativity differences between the atoms and the molecule's geometry. If the geometry supports some molecular *asymmetry*, and if there are electronegativity differences, you most likely have a polar molecule.

Whenever you think of molecules being polar versus nonpolar, you will be able to figure out if they will *like each other* in a solution. Any molecule dissolving in water, which is polar, must itself be polar. Remember the phrase: *like dissolves like.* Polar and polar will be fine when mixed together, while nonpolar and polar do not mix. In the same way, two nonpolar molecules are fine when mixed together. This is the reason why oil (nonpolar) and water (polar) do not mix.

What are amphipathic molecules?

Amphipathic molecules are usually very large, confusing structures. A part of it will clearly be nonpolar, while another will be polar. A classic example of this type of molecule is the phospholipid. These are the molecules making up a big part of the cell membrane of all cells on earth. The cell membrane is an interesting sandwich called a *bilayer*. A phospholipid bilayer *shows* its polar water-loving or *hydrophilic* ends to the outside world (where it is watery) but maintains an internal sandwich filling of the water-hating or *hydrophobic* ends. This image shows you what a phospholipid looks like:

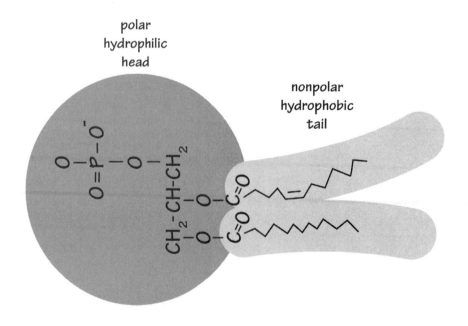

In a cell membrane, the tails all huddle together in the middle of two outside sheets of polar heads, where, in living things, proteins and other lipids float around on what biologists call the *lipid raft*. It looks like this:

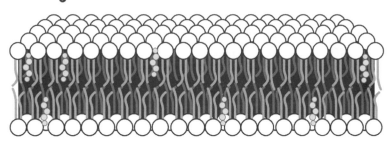

bilayer sheet

> **Did you know?** The soap you use in everyday life is made from amphipathic molecules. These are molecules that mix with and trap the grease on your hands and dishes, collecting it in balls called "micelles." With the grease safely tucked away inside the micelle, you can just use water to wash the grease away to keep things clean.

Let's Wrap This Up

The covalent bond is more of a sharing experience between two atoms, although the sharing will never be completely equal unless the atoms themselves are the same. If not, one atom will pull the electron being shared toward itself. Look for the more electronegative atom to be greedier in wanting the valence electron.

There can be single, double, or triple bonds in covalent bonding. The sigma bond will always be stronger because the orbitals overlap directly; the pi bond is not as strong because the orbitals just graze each other from the side. An aromatic compound and resonance molecules will involve electrons being indecisive about where to go, moving back and forth between double and single bonds.

Polarity is important to understand in chemistry. A nonpolar substance will be hydrophobic or *water-hating*, while a polar substance will love water and is said to be hydrophilic. Amphipathic molecules tend to be large and have both polar and nonpolar components.

CHAPTER 7:

OTHER BOND TYPES

There are other types of bonds besides ionic and covalent bonds. Before we talk about these, you should know something about bond strength. Clearly, some bonds are stronger than others. It turns out that you can predict the strength of a bond between two atoms, and, if you feel like you don't want to do this, there are tables you can find that will tell how strong the bond will be.

Why would this be important? In many cases, it might not be, but if you want to know what two substrates in a reaction will do, you can see if a bond between two atoms in any substrate is weak enough to be pulled off as part of the reaction. This leads us to the concept of bond energy.

Bond energy is the amount of energy you would need to break any covalent bond. The bond energy will depend on several things. It certainly depends on which atoms/elements you are dealing with, but it also depends on the circumstances. A single bond between hydrogen and carbon (the C-H bond) is not the same in all molecules. If other bonds in the molecule have already been broken, this could affect the bond energy in the C-H bond you are trying to break.

While it is not hard and fast, you can generally say that the order of bond strength between the different bond types is this:

Ionic bonds > Covalent bonds > Hydrogen bonds > Van der Waals forces > London dispersion forces

We have not yet talked about hydrogen bonds, van der Waals forces, or London dispersion forces. These are so weak in some cases that the latter two aren't even called bonds. Instead, they are forces or attractions between a variety of atoms.

Hydrogen bonds

Hydrogen bonds must, of course, involve a hydrogen atom and some other atom. It can occur between two separate molecules or between atoms in the same (usually larger) molecule. If you look at the electronegativity of hydrogen, you'll see that it is 2.2, which is in the middle of the pack. This means that it will never form a true ionic bond with anything but it has a decent ability to attract other atoms. Common atoms you'll see linked to hydrogen in this type of bonding or attraction are oxygen, hydrogen, and fluorine.

How does this work? In water, or H_2O, a great deal of hydrogen bonding is going on. If you could take a very close look, you would see these types of interactions:

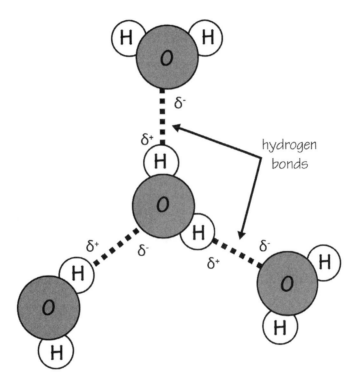

See how there are attractions between the hydrogen and oxygen atoms _between_ water molecules? It's because of the little bit of magnetism or dipole moments in the water molecules. As the molecules align themselves, they set up a situation where hydrogen and oxygen atoms stay close to one another in a liquid-water situation. It's what makes water have many of its properties, like a high melting and boiling point (compared to other molecules of the same size).

What about ice and hydrogen bonding? There is hydrogen bonding here too, but the arrangement of molecules is different. The way water molecules in ice are arranged, the molecules are actually further apart than they are with liquid water. In short, this leads to a decreased density of ice compared to water and is exactly why ice is less dense than water. You can see this clearly in this image:

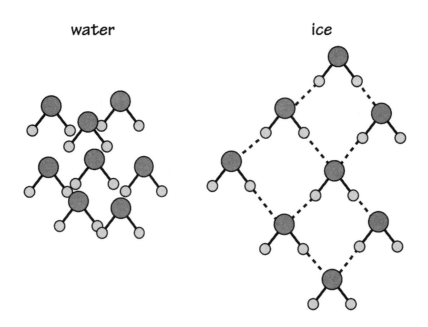

In chemistry, this density property of ice is very unusual in most small molecules, yet it is the very reason we have life on earth. What would have happened to ancient life (or even modern aquatic life) if ice sunk to the bottom and eventually filled an entire lake or pond?

Hydrogen in any bond with an electronegative atom will have that atom draw the hydrogen's electron away from it. This creates a slight positivity on the hydrogen atom. We call this the hydrogen bond donor. ***NOTE: It doesn't really donate anything. It just makes the hydrogen atom more positive electrically so it will be attracted to some other electronegative atom.***

There is also a hydrogen bond acceptor. The hydrogen atom that has been made positive now needs to attract to a hydrogen bond acceptor. This is often a highly electronegative atom like oxygen, fluorine, or nitrogen. You need to understand that the hydrogen atom is now attracted to the lone pair of electrons floating around these electronegative atoms. The more electronegative an atom is, the greater its attraction will be to this hydrogen atom.

Hydrogen bonding is extremely important in biochemistry and the biology of living things. Do you remember that the DNA molecule is a double helix? It consists of two strands of matching base pairs that are themselves attached to each other through hydrogen bonding. It would be impossible to have a stable double helix without hydrogen bonds extending from one end of the DNA strand to the other. Because hydrogen bonding is relatively weak, however, the strands can unzip when needed in order to allow the DNA to be replicated as part of its everyday activities.

Another place where hydrogen bonding is extremely important is in protein structure. Proteins are basically long lines of amino acids. They would work very well if they didn't have a unique shape. As you will see later, there are many things that can cause this unique shape. One of these is hydrogen bonding between different amino acids in the polypeptide or protein chain.

Van der Waals forces

As we have discussed, van der Waals forces can also result from an attraction between different neutral molecules. How does this work? We know that van der Waals forces work in gases, liquids, and solids. In 1873, a physicist named Johannes van der Waals was curious about attractions he perceived in gaseous molecules that were neutral in electric charge. He also found that solids could have van der Waals forces, which led to lower melting points than he would have otherwise predicted. This is why he proposed the idea of some attractive force going on.

To be sure, these forces are relatively weak, but they can have powerful effects. The idea behind them is that other molecules that do not contain hydrogen will also have dipole moments. These molecules will also be attracted to other molecules with dipole moments, resulting in a weak attractive force between them. As with hydrogen bonding, you can think of these dipole moments as being relatively permanent and fixed as part of the molecule's structure. All of this can add up so that you'll see significant interactions between all the different molecules in any given collection of gas, solid, or liquid. You can think of van der Waals forces as a type of molecular static electricity. This image shows you how it works:

van der waals' forces (VDW) diagram

\+ positive nucleus
\- negative charged electron cloud

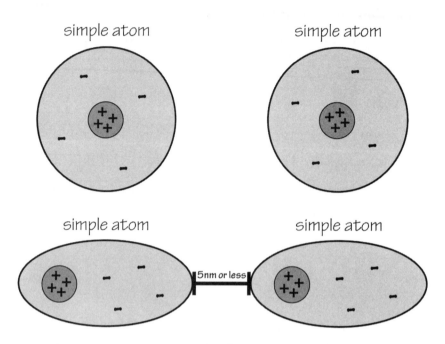

simple atom   simple atom

simple atom   simple atom

5nm or less

when two atoms come within 5 nanometers of each other,
there will be a slight interaction between them,
thus causing polarity and a slight attraction

You can see in this image that even though atoms are supposed to have a symmetric cloud of electrons around them, this is not the case, leaving the electron cloud somewhat lopsided if other atoms are near it.

Did you know? Van der Waals forces can be extremely powerful. Have you ever wondered how geckos stick to the ceiling and walls around them? Their pads are not sticky at all. Scientists have discovered that these geckos are held up by van der Waals forces existing between the task of their feet and the molecules in the walls and ceiling they hang from. Weird, isn't it?

London Dispersion Forces

London dispersion forces are the weakest of all forces between atoms. To be fair, London dispersion forces are a type of van der Waals force. Unfortunately, they are harder to understand. If you think of the electron cloud around an atom as being symmetric some of the time and asymmetric or lopsided other times, it makes more sense. The odds are that some of the time, the electron cloud will be lopsided. When this happens, there will be a tiny dipole moment within that electron cloud. It looks a lot like this:

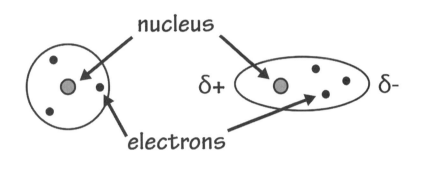

symmetrical distribution   unsymmetrical distribution

While this looks a lot like the van der Waals forces we just discussed, the key feature here is that the dipole moment is temporary in London dispersion forces. This means that very inert substances like argon can have an attraction to other argon atoms, but only if the temperature is very cold and argon becomes liquefied. As you can imagine, larger atoms with many electrons will be more wobbly and can exert a greater London dispersion force on another atom compared to small atoms.

How would you notice this? If you consider liquid argon and liquid helium together, you can see this better. Argon and helium are both inert noble gases; however, argon is much bigger. Because of this, liquid argon sticks together better, and it takes more energy to boil into a gas. Liquid argon boils at 87 degrees Kelvin; however, its helium counterpart boils at just one degree Kelvin. The reason for this is solely because of the London dispersion forces being greater in liquid argon.

You can also see this in liquid nitrogen, commonly used in all sorts of scientific and medical circles. Without London dispersion forces, it would be impossible to even liquefy this gas. Basically, these forces involve static electricity in the same way as with van der Waals forces. The difference is that the static electricity happens sheerly by random chance and because of the electron cloud's temporary lopsidedness around the atom.

Let's Wrap This Up

In this chapter, you studied some of the weaker bonds in chemistry. Of these, hydrogen bonding is the most common and significant in areas of chemistry like organic chemistry and biochemistry. Life on earth could not exist without this important type of bond.

Van der Waals forces and London dispersion forces are somewhat confusing because they don't represent real bonds. Instead, these are forces that exist between atoms and molecules based on dipole moments that may be permanent (as in van der Waals forces) or transient (as in London dispersion forces). While these are weak forces, just ask any gecko how important they really are.

SECTION 4:
CHEMICAL REACTIONS

It's totally fine to talk all day about atoms and molecules; however, the real action comes when these substances interact with one another. In truth, molecules react with one another all the time, even outside of a chemistry lab. Consider your nice vehicle sitting in the parking lot. Is it as shiny and nice as it used to be? Does it have some rust? If so, the rust you see is actually a chemical reaction happening spontaneously in nature. We will talk about how this reaction happens later.

In this chapter, we will talk about how you go about writing chemical equations. It is okay to say "water and salt A mix together to make salts B and salt C." While the chemist next to you might understand this, this is not the proper way to write a chemical reaction. Even when you know how to write the reaction, you need to balance the equation. Most of the time, balancing is easy if you pay attention.

Then we'll talk about the practical part. What do you do if you want to make 100 grams of a salt product? How much substrate for *reactants* do you need? Practically speaking, it would be impossible to put together two reactants in exactly the right amount to make exactly 100 grams of the salt product you want. There will always be a *limiting reagent* that will be used up completely, with some of the other reactants left over.

There are several different kinds of reactions you need to learn about. By the end of the section, you will know the different kinds of chemical reactions and be able to identify them on sight alone. It's not the amazing feat you might imagine it to be. Let's get started.

CHAPTER 8:

CHEMICAL EQUATIONS

This chapter looks at chemical equations and how they are written. By now, hopefully, you will be able to look at the symbol for any element and know what the old name really is. You will need this knowledge to be able to write chemical equations. As you will see, there are a few other notations that help make it clear what you are talking about when you write your equations.

Formulae and Symbolic Representation

Besides the atomic abbreviations themselves, you need to know a few other things when writing chemical equations. First, all equations are written with the reactants or substrates on the left-hand side and the end products or *products* on the right-hand side.

In between these two halves, things can get interesting. Ideally, you would write an arrow going from the left to the right. This makes sense, right? In chemistry, however, it doesn't make sense. When you write an arrow that goes from left to right, the implication is that the reaction goes mostly, if not completely, in that direction. In reality, few reactions actually go this way. This leads to a complicated mess of arrows you need to be able to interpret. Let's try to make sense of them.

1. **Writing a forward arrow**: This is your typical reaction arrow. What you mean to say is that A + B makes C + D. A typical reaction might look like this:

$$A + B \longrightarrow C + D$$

2. **Writing an equilibrium arrow:** You will write an equilibrium arrow whenever the reaction goes both ways. In the event that a reaction goes more in one direction than another, you would simply make that arrow longer, as shown:

$$A + B \rightleftharpoons C + D \qquad \text{Reversible reaction}$$

$$A + B \rightleftharpoons C + D \qquad \text{Mostly favors products}$$

$$A + B \rightleftharpoons C + D \qquad \text{Mostly favors reactants}$$

3. **Writing the resonance arrow:** You may not have to use the resonance arrow very much. This is only used when writing the inter-conversion between two resonance forms. It looks like this:

4. **Writing an arrow with a dash:** this is the arrow you write when you are simply suggesting the possibility that the reactants might become products but do not know how this would occur. It looks like this:

$$A + B \dashrightarrow[\text{conditions?}] C + D$$

(how can these reactants
become these products?)

5. **Writing a curved arrow:** A curved arrow in chemistry usually means you are describing the movement of a pair of electrons. It is not generally part of an equation unless you wish to show this step. It looks like this:

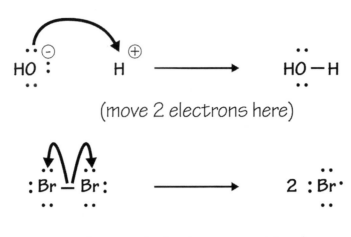

(move 2 electrons here)

(move 1 electron at a time)

6. **The meaning of a broken arrow:** A broken arrow indicates any reaction that does not work or is expected not to work if tested. You would often see it look like this:

$$A + B \xslashed{} C + D$$

$$A + B \xslashed{} C + D$$

Other things you should know are the abbreviations for water (aq), solid (s), liquid (l), and gas (g). Once you know these things, you will be able to write an accurate representation of a chemical reaction. Let's look at a basic reaction:

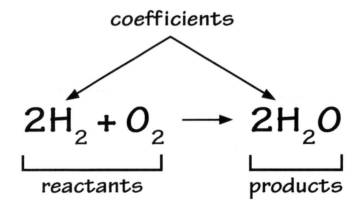

The reaction is simple. Hydrogen gas and oxygen mix together to make water. The number 2 before hydrogen gas and water is called the coefficient. Water doesn't need it because the coefficient is 1 (which does not need to be written down). The arrow is generally written, so you can assume the reaction is moving forward (but it's not a guarantee).

The coefficient tells you the molar ratio involved in the reaction but nothing about how much of each substance you would add in a laboratory. We'll talk more about how to do this later. It simply tells you how many moles of one substance you'd add to a certain number of moles of another substance to get the end products.

To get fancier and more specific about your equation, you can add qualifiers to say the state the substance is in during the reaction. The example shown here tells you these states in parentheses. Note that here, everything is in its gaseous state, so you can imagine the temperature of the reaction happens above the boiling point of water:

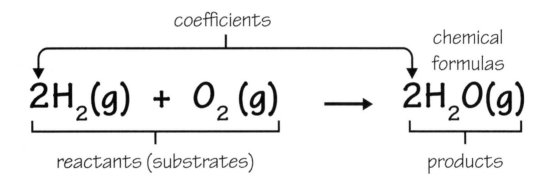

In some cases, you will need to write whether or not energy is necessary for the reaction. The symbol delta (Δ) is used above the reaction arrow to show this. Also, if you need to add light energy to the equation, you will indicate this by writing the symbol *hv*. The image shown tells you whether heat must be added to the system. Technically, you can say how much heat you need to apply to the reaction, as you can see by the second equation:

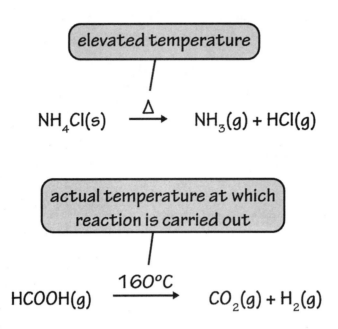

Stoichiometry and Balancing

Writing the equation is one thing; writing one that is balanced is altogether different. The study of balancing equations is called stoichiometry. The idea behind it is that mole-for-mole, the reaction must proceed so you don't magically create an atom of anything in a reaction (or destroy one either).

In order to balance the equation, you need to look at each atom of each element on both sides of the equation. Every atom should be of the same number, even if it turns up as a different molecule on the opposite side. The chemical equations above are completely balanced.

Let's say you know the reactants and products in a chemical reaction but do not have a balanced equation. Start by writing down what you do know:

$$CH4 + Cl2 \rightarrow CCl4 + HCl$$

What you just wrote would be that methane and chlorine gas go to make carbon tetrachloride and hydrochloric acid. What you need now is to balance this equation. The next step is to add the number of atoms of each element on either side of the equation:

- Reactants (left side): Carbon-1, Hydrogen-4, Chlorine-2
- Products (right side): Carbon-1, Hydrogen-1, Chlorine-5

Well, this is a problem, isn't it? Carbon is perfect, but both hydrogen and chlorine are off. How do you correct this? Start by fixing the hydrogen atoms. You need to have enough on both sides to match the total hydrogen atoms on each side. Add 4 to the righthand side to get a matched set. This changes the equation, which is still unbalanced, to look like this:

$$CH4 + Cl2 \rightarrow CCl4 + 4HCl$$

Now, you have 2 chlorines on the left and 8 on the right. Can you see what needs to be done next? By changing the coefficient on the chlorine gas (Cl2) molecule, you will then have a balanced equation:

$$CH4 + 4Cl2 \rightarrow CCl4 + 4HCl$$

The equation is now perfectly balanced. To be fair, balancing is not always this straightforward. For this reason, you should practice a few of these, and if you get stuck, there are websites you can use to check your work (or do it for you!). Remember the Law of Conservation of Mass, which says that matter cannot be created or destroyed. What this means for you and in writing chemical equations is that every equation you write must be totally balanced.

Once you've got this down, it is a simple matter to calculate the molar ratio of anything you wish in the reaction. The molar ratio tells you how many moles of something you'll get if you add a certain number of moles of reactant to the system. In the above equation, you simply have to take any two molecules and divide their coefficients. With regard to HCl and Chlorine gas (Cl2), the molar ratio is 1/4. If you wanted to make a mole of hydrochloric acid, for example, you would need to add 4 moles of chlorine gas.

This seems easy, but you still do not know exactly how much gas you would need to add in order to get a certain amount of HCl at the end of the reaction (assuming the reaction goes to completion without difficulty). Let's look at this thorny problem in practical chemistry.

Problem: You need 100 grams of HCl. How much chlorine gas would you need to have on hand to accomplish this, given this balanced reaction:

$$CH4+4Cl2 \rightarrow CCl4+4HCl$$

You would now need to determine how many moles of HCl make up 100 grams. Look up the atomic masses for hydrogen and chlorine and add them. This is the molar mass for HCl.

Substance	Atomic or Molar Mass
Hydrogen	1.008 amu (g/mol)
Chlorine	34.968 amu (g/mol)
Hydrochloric acid (HCl)	35.967 g/mole

Next, you do the calculations:

$$100g\left(\frac{mol}{35.967g}\right) = 2.78 \text{ mole}$$

Perfect! You already know the molar ratio in this equation is 1:1 Chlorine gas: Hydrochloric acid. This obviously means you'll need the same number of moles of chlorine gas (Cl_2) to add on the left-hand side. If the molar mass of chlorine gas is 71.934 g/mole (and it is!), you would multiply this number with 2.78 moles to get a total of 199.98 grams of chlorine gas (how much this is in terms of volume would depend on the pressure and temperature of the system).

Limiting Reagent

The limiting reagent in any chemical reaction system is the reactant that will get used up in your reaction. It is easiest to do when there are just two reagents, but it can be done in any system. You would need to know how much of each reagent you've added, the molar masses of each, and the coefficients (so you can calculate the molar ratio).

In the above equation, let's say you decide to add 100 grams of methane. Is it enough to use up all the chlorine gas you have? If not, this would be the limiting reagent. You would first calculate the molar mass of methane or CH_4. Hydrogen adds 1.008 x 4 or 4.032 grams per mole to the molar mass, while carbon adds an additional 12.01 grams per mole. The total molar mass is 16.042 grams per mole. Your 100 grams of methane is a total of 6.23 moles.

The difference in this calculation compared to the one we just did is that the molar ratio is 4:1 between chlorine gas and methane. For every mole of chlorine gas, you need just 1/4 the number of moles of methane. If you are adding 2.78 moles of chlorine gas, you would only need a quarter of that, or 0.695 moles. Doing your calculations, you see how you have nearly 10 times the number of moles you need. You would only have needed to add 11.15 grams (not 100 grams!) if you wanted to use it up completely. In this case, the chlorine gas is the limiting reagent; it will be used up, and you will have lots of methane leftover. In fact, you will have added 88.85 grams too much methane.

In some cases, you want to add enough of something in the reaction in order to use it up completely, especially if it would contaminate the end products in some way or be hard to get rid of when you *clean up* the end product afterward. You might also choose to limit the amount of a more precious reagent so as to reduce wastage. In any event, these types of calculations help you put a practical spin on your chemical reactions in the lab.

Let's Wrap This Up

As you can see, writing and interpreting chemical reactions correctly will help you make sense of chemistry in ways you can't do in any other convenient way. Once you know what reaction you are trying to do, you can simplify the *story* of the reaction by writing it out in the form of a simple equation.

Balancing the equation is essential if you want to be accurate about what is happening. In fact, it is very hard to decide how to perform the experiment practically if you don't know the molar ratios involved. Remember, atoms and molecules don't care much about size in their interactions with one another. Instead, it's the molar ratios of each reactant that are important. Use what you know to determine practically how much of each reagent/reactant you need in your experiment.

CHAPTER 9:

TYPES OF CHEMICAL REACTIONS

You may think that all chemical reactions are created the same. After you read this chapter, you will see that this is not the case; you should also be able to look at a chemical equation and know how to say what type of reaction you are dealing with.

At the end of the chapter, we will discuss a particular type of reaction, known as the redox reaction. In reality, this will never be just a single reaction; it will instead involve a pair of reactions. One will be called an oxidation reaction; the other is a reduction reaction (which explains the name *redox*). These specifically involve exchanges of electrons in a series of reactions. As you already know, if one part involves donating an electron, you need another part to accept it. In chemistry, giving an electron away into space isn't practical and just doesn't take place in your average chemistry beaker.

Summary of Reaction Types

These are not terribly difficult to understand. They can be divided into reactions that create molecules, those that break them down, and several others. We will talk about a few of these in detail afterward.

- *Combination reactions*—these build a molecule from smaller molecules or atoms. Some call these synthesis reactions. They are easy to see because you'll have fewer products than you have reactants. A general reaction of this nature would look like this: $A + B \rightarrow AB$. A more specific reaction of this type would be something like $2Na + Cl_2 \rightarrow 2NaCl$.

- **Decomposition reactions**—these are not like decomposing flesh or anything creepy at all. Instead, they are the opposite of a combination reaction. There will be more end products than reactants because one or more compound is broken down. If something decomposes from heat application, it is called a thermal decomposition reaction. It might look like this: AB → A + B. A real-life application would be this: $CaCO_3$ → CaO + CO_2.

- **Precipitation reactions**—these are dramatic because they involve mixing two solutions of salts that ultimately combine to make two other salts. One of these salts has properties that make it insoluble in water. It precipitates out into the solution, where you would then be able to remove the liquid and dry out the solid part, called the precipitate. These reactions often go to completion more than others because the precipitate essentially leaves the picture, so the chance of any reverse reacting going on is very low. Here is a real-life example: $NaCl(aq)$ + $AgNO_3(aq)$ → $AgCl(s)$ + $NaNO_3(aq)$. Notice that the $AgCl$ is a solid that will precipitate out of the solution.

- **Neutralization reactions**—these are acid/base reactions where acids and bases interact to make a salt and water. In short, an acid would be *acidic*, while a base would be *basic* or *alkaline*. When they mix together, they neutralize the pH of the water they are dissolved in. Very simply, they look like this: Acid + Base → Salt + Water. As you will see, water is not just a bystander; it is an end product.

- **Combustion reactions**—these always involve oxygen and always give off carbon dioxide and water. These are exactly what they sound like; they involve combustion and give off heat. Basically, they look somewhat like this: A + O_2 → H_2O + CO_2.

- **Displacement reactions**—these are simply the mixing and matching of elements in a reaction. You might also call this a substitution reaction. You will sometimes see these looking like this: A + BC → AC + B. What this means is that you've mixed molecules when one element is so reactive that it displaces the element in the other molecule. Most likely, it is a situation where one atom is far greedier than another, snatching off the other atom in order to take its place. Here is a real-life example: Zn + $CuSO_4$ → $ZnSO_4$ + Cu.

- **Double displacement reactions**—these are reactions where certain ions get exchanged to make two completely unique salts or compounds. It's a lot like switching dance partners at a dance and generally looks like this: XY + ZA → XZ + YA. Some call this a metathesis reaction; a real-life example would look like this: BBaCl2 + Na2SO4 → BaSO4 + 2NaCl.

This is a pictorial representation of what this tends to look like:

combination reaction

$$A + B \rightarrow AB$$

decomposition reaction

$$Cl\,Na \rightarrow Cl + Na$$

$$AB \rightarrow A + B$$

combustion reaction

$$CH + O_2 \rightarrow CO_2 + H_2O$$

neutralization reaction

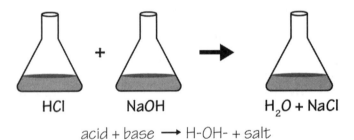

HCl   NaOH   H₂O + NaCl

acid + base ⟶ H-OH- + salt

double displacement reaction

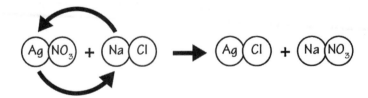

$$Ag\,NO_3 + Na\,Cl \rightarrow Ag\,Cl + Na\,NO_3$$

Redox Reactions

Redox reactions change the oxidation number of an atom. What the heck is an oxidation number, anyway? Before we proceed, let's nail down this thorny definition. This number is the total number of electrons any atom either loses or gains as part of making a chemical bond. You can assign an oxidation number to any atom fairly simply because it is _the charge any atom would have if it became an ion._

Let's say you have a molecule of iron oxide or hematite, which is Fe2O3 (Fe_2O_3). Iron, or Fe, in this case, has an oxidation number of +3 because it has three spots for electrons it needs to make an ionic bond. Oxygen has an oxidation number of -2 because it wants to donate two electrons to the bond. As you can imagine, if a molecule is just an ordinary one, it will be neutral once you add up the oxidation numbers.

Here are some tricks you might need to get started:

- All single neutral atoms have an oxidation number of zero.
- All molecules with just one atom in them have an oxidation number of zero (including large ones like P_4 and S_8).
- All ions have an oxidation number the same as their charge.
- Hydrogen ions have a +1 oxidation number if combined with any nonmetal (think CH4, H2O, or NH3). The oxidation number is -1 if combined with a metal (think CaH2 or NaH).
- Group 1A atoms (lithium, potassium, and sodium, for example) have an oxidation number of +1 in any compound (like Na2S).
- Group IIA atoms (magnesium, calcium, etc.) have an oxidation number of +2 in any compound (like CaCO2).
- Expect oxygen to have an oxidation number of -2 unless it is combined only with itself or in any O-O bond.
- The group VIIA atoms have a -1 oxidation number when in compounds like HCl or AlF3.
- Iron and related atoms have an oxidation number equal to the number in parentheses after them in a compound (such as Iron (II) chloride). This will be a positive number.
- The sum of all oxidation numbers will be zero if the molecule itself is zero.

In redox reactions, the oxidation number changes because electrons are passed from one chemical substance to another. It happens in this reaction:

$$2\,S_2O_3{}^{2-}(aq) + I_2(aq) \rightarrow S_4O_6{}^{2-}(aq) + 2\,I^-(aq)$$

Iodine goes from an oxidation number of zero on the lefthand side to -1 on the righthand side. Sulfur goes from +2 to +2.5 from left to right. Let's look at the sulfur molecule:

- **$S_2O_3{}^{2-}$:** Because oxygen is -2 and there are 3 of them, this would be a total of -6. If this were a neutral compound, the oxidation number of sulfur would have to be +3. But the molecule is negatively charged, so you need to subtract this number to get a -4 total contribution. As there are 2 sulfur atoms, each contributes +2 to the molecule. Added up, you get +4 from sulfur and -6 from oxygen, which is why the whole thing has a -2 charge.
- **$S_4O_6{}^{2-}$:** Because oxygen is still -2, its contribution is -12. Subtract the ionic charge of -2 to get -10. Divide this by 4, as there are four sulfur atoms, to get an oxidation number of +2.5.

This redox reaction has two parts: oxidation and reduction. What does this mean? Here is the basic definition:

- **Oxidation = loss of electrons (gain of oxidation number)**
- **Reduction = gain of electrons (loss of oxidation number)**

What this means is that you need to look at the oxidation number. If it is *reduced*, or lessened, this is reduction. If it is gained, or increased, this is oxidation. Hopefully, this image helps clear things up visually for you:

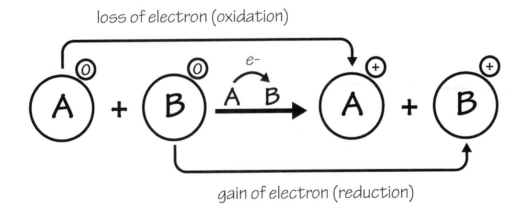

In a redox reaction, the entire thing must be balanced. If an electron is gained by one atom (reducing its oxidation number by x amount), another atom must have given an electron (with its own oxidation number increased by the same x amount).You can now see where many reactions can be redox reactions: decomposition, composition, and displacement reactions. You need to look carefully at the molecule to decide the oxidation numbers on both sides of the equation in order to see if a redox reaction has occurred. You can also cheat and use an online oxidation number calculator.

What are Oxidizing and Reducing Agents?

Oxidizers or oxidizing agents are molecules, atoms, or ions that love to gain electrons so they can be reduced themselves. They need to oxidize something in order to do this. Reducing agents like to get rid of electrons so as to be oxidized. When they do this, they must reduce something else. You should know the major oxidizing and reducing agents:

- **Oxidizing agents:** These include many things with oxygen in them or any of the halogens. You can look at things like O_2, O_3, $KmnO_4$, metal oxides like CuO or MgO, and fluorine. You can imagine that fluorine is the strongest oxidizing agent because it is so electronegative. It wants electrons so badly, it will snatch one from anywhere.
- **Reducing agents:** These include all metals (like Fe, Zn, or Na), hydrogen, phosphorus, sulfur, acids containing hydrogen (like HBr or HCl), metal hydrides (metals that bind to hydrogen), and any element in its least oxidation state (like iron (II)). Lithium and cesium are the strongest reducing agents in chemistry.

You should know that some things are either oxidizing or reducing agents, such as H_2SO_4, SO_2, and H_2O_2.

Let's Wrap This Up

The different types of reactions aren't very important to really memorize; the idea is to show you that many kinds of reactions can occur in chemistry. You should be able to recognize redox reactions, however. Memorize what identifies oxidation and what is reduction; remember that it is impossible to have reduction without oxidation (and vice versa).

SECTION 5:
THERMODYNAMICS AND ELECTROCHEMISTRY

While electrochemistry and thermodynamics seem to be two of the more boring topics in all of chemistry, understanding these topics will help you feel more confident in your ability to grasp chemistry. Thermodynamics is the more important of the two because thermodynamics explains a lot of what goes on in chemistry—even on a tiny scale. Chemical reactions always follow the laws of thermodynamics. You will be able to see after reading this exactly why some chemical reactions happen spontaneously, just as others don't.

Electrochemistry is not used as much in regular chemistry labs, but you can learn important chemical principles by studying this concept. Oxidation reactions leading to corrosion of metals are an important topic to get a handle on; it is a common phenomenon best explained when you know the chemistry behind it.

CHAPTER 10:

THERMODYNAMICS
AND EQUILIBRIUM

Thermodynamics applies to everything in nature. Once you know the details, you will see how to apply these laws to chemical principles. You will also be able to determine whether or not a reaction will proceed forward and to what degree it will do this, if at all.

Laws of Thermodynamics

It took about a century in the mid-1800s to early 1900s to come up with the laws of thermodynamics, which describe what we know about heat and energy. The only major mistake they made was that they felt they had the trifecta of three perfect laws before someone came up with a fourth law. It didn't make sense to have this last law be called *number four* because it logically preceded the other laws, so it had to be called the zeroth law. Let's look at what these laws are trying to say about physics and chemistry:

- **Zeroth Law of Thermodynamics**—this is actually the last law named. It was considered too obvious at first to be called a law, until Robert Fowler, a British physicist, proposed it. This law states that if two physical bodies are the same temperature and in equilibrium with one another, and if one of these is in equilibrium with a third body, then all three are in equilibrium. You can see why this one is kind of obvious.

- **First Law of Thermodynamics**—this means that the increase in energy you'll see in any system is the temperature increase plus any work done on the system. Heat is energy, so it must be conserved in some way, even if it is turned into another form.

- **Second Law of Thermodynamics**—this is a law stating that you can't transfer any energy from a system with lower energy into one with higher energy without adding something energetic to the system. It explains why you can cool a room or home but that it costs electrical energy to do this. It is the heat equivalent of why a ball won't roll up a hill without adding energy. In the same way, chemical reactions do not happen uphill (to higher energy states) without applying energy.

- **Third Law of Thermodynamics**—this law can be described in many ways. The focus is on entropy, which is a measure of disorder in any physical system. The object with the least entropy would be a pure crystal sitting at absolute zero. Of course, it is impossible to have a pure crystal or to reach absolute zero in any real-life situation. The idea is that if a perfect crystal existed at this temperature, it would have no entropy or disorder because the atoms would be completely immobile. You can think of entropy like what would happen if you put a toddler into a clean kitchen and told him to make himself a snack. By the end of the time, there would certainly be disorder there. In chemical systems, the tendency would also be toward greater entropy or more disorder unless energy reverses this process. _Motion equals disorder in most physical systems where energy isn't applied to reverse this._

Enthalpy and Entropy

We should take this opportunity to look more closely at enthalpy and entropy. Enthalpy is often equated with heat, which is inaccurate. In the same way, heat and temperature are not the same things. Heat is a concept, while temperature is a way of quantifying heat, so it makes sense to us.

The term _enthalpy_ means, in Greek, to put heat into something. In specific terms, enthalpy is related to heat, energy, and pressure. It is related to energy but really isn't the same thing at all. One way to describe enthalpy is to take a system under unchanging pressure and change the substances in some way. If you do this, you will add or subtract heat, AND you will add or subtract work to change the substance. _This combination of heat plus work is equal to enthalpy._

You can also apply enthalpy to a gaseous system. If you increase the heat, you will increase the energy of the system without changing its pressure by trapping the gas. You might also add work to the system to expand the gas. This expansion of gas is how many engines and piston systems work.

There is a calculation used to describe enthalpy. It is described as the internal energy of a system plus pressure multiplied by volume. It looks like this:

$$H = E = Pv$$

Enthalpy applies to chemical systems as well as physical systems. In chemistry, it is not uncommon for the end products in a reaction to be colder or warmer than they were before the reaction. Heat will flow out of the system until it equilibrates with its surroundings. If you can keep this from happening and also keep the pressure the same, the temperature change will say a lot about what happened to the enthalpy of the situation (because it relates to the heat change directly).

For example, if you have a reaction that burns up the substrates or gives off a great deal of heat, you can not only say that the enthalpy of the substance is the same, but you can also say that the enthalpy of the substance you have burned is now less. The lost enthalpy went into the surrounding air as heat (that heated the air around it). In addition, if you can quantitate the heat given off (usually in kilojoules or joules), you can actually say how many kilojoules of enthalpy were in the original substance.

What this means is that a reaction that gives off heat is said to lose enthalpy, and you will report it as a number like this: ΔH = −100 kJ. If you have a reaction that actually needs heat or one where the end products are colder after the reaction is over, you now have a positive enthalpy situation because work has been put into the reaction. This work, as you know, counts as part of enthalpy. You could write the reaction like this: ΔH = +100 kJ.

Chemical reactions that give off heat are called exothermic reactions. Those that become cooler after the reaction are called endothermic reactions. You will now be able to tell if a reaction is endothermic or exothermic by the delta H (ΔH) sign. If it is positive, the reaction is endothermic. If it has a delta H (ΔH), the reaction is exothermic.

Specific Heat

The specific heat of a substance is a value given to some material based on several factors. The measurement of the specific heat is in *joules per gram-degree*. The specific heat of water is defined as 1 calorie per gram degree Celsius, which is 4.186 joules per gram degree Celsius. What this means is that you have to add 1 calorie to a single gram of water in order to raise it 1 degree Celsius. `

Water actually has a very high specific heat compared to other molecules of a similar size. This is because there are so many hydrogen bonds compared to other molecules that the specific gravity is higher than it otherwise would be. There are tables you can use to look up the specific gravity of other substances. For example, vegetable oil has a specific heat of just 2.0 joules per gram degree Celsius. This is less than half of the specific heat of water. The specific heat of anything is constant and does not change.

Entropy

Entropy, or *disorder*, is the amount of energy in any substance that cannot do work. Remember that things with enthalpy will do work, but any entropy in the substance won't perform any job requiring energy. Suppose you think of a piece of paper that you burn. Once burned, you won't have any ability to use the burned fragments and ashes. These latter objects will not perform work; they are too disordered.

Entropy can mean randomness in chemistry. Random molecules in gaseous form have a great deal more entropy than the same gas condensed into solid form by cooling it enough. Entropy can never decrease by itself, according to the third law of thermodynamics. You need to add energy to do this. It is like your living room. It doesn't take much to mess it up, but it can be clean again, if you put some physical work or energy into putting it back in order.

Potential and Gibbs Free Energy

According to the second law of thermodynamics, entropy will increase in any process that happens spontaneously. Other reactions that need added energy will have decreased entropy of the end products. If you want to quantify these things further, you can measure the enthalpy of the substrates or reactants as well as the enthalpy of the end products. The difference between these two things is called the Gibbs free energy.

The initial for Gibbs free energy is G. If this number is negative, the reaction is considered to be spontaneous. Each item has a known enthalpy level, so you can actually calculate the difference between the two sides of the reaction.

This handy table will help you decide if a reaction will be spontaneous or not. As you'll see, spontaneity is sometimes based on the temperature of the reaction system:

Change in Enthalpy	Change in Entropy	Gibbs Free Energy	Spontaneous?
Positive	Positive	Depends on temperature	Only if the temperature is high
Negative	Positive	Negative	Always
Negative	Negative	Depends on temperature	Only if the temperature is low
Positive	Negative	Positive	Never

The Gibbs free energy is related to what we call the **equilibrium constant.** This will be talked about next. However, it's safe to say that you can use the Gibbs free energy to say whether or not a reaction will happen. Here are some tricks you should know:

- A large negative ΔG means that the reaction is spontaneous and will go to completion. The equilibrium constant K will be high to indicate a nearly complete reaction.
- Any reaction with a positive ΔG will not be favorable and will have a small equilibrium constant.
- If you see that the ΔG is zero, the reaction will be at complete equilibrium.
- There is more than one ΔG you might run into. The term ΔG^o is the free energy change done in standard conditions (which is 1 molar concentration, one atmosphere, and 25 degrees Celsius). If you just see a ΔG, it doesn't indicate a standard state and could be at any state or condition.

Equilibrium Constant

It would be nice if all reactions went in the forward direction to completion. This rarely happens, however. As you mix reactants and products in water, for example, they will sit there in the same soup as the reactions happen. At first, there will just be reactants and no products. Then products build up into the mix. This opens up the door to the possibility that the products will react themselves, becoming reactants again. These are called reversible reactions.

Equilibrium happens eventually. What this means is that the forward rate and the reverse rate are the same, and no further change in the reaction substances occurs. It can also be called *steady state*. It doesn't mean that nothing is happening; it only means that the concentrations of everything in the reaction are stable.

Since few reactions actually go 100 percent to completion, you need to have some way of determining just how far a reaction will go. This is what the equilibrium constant is all about. High equilibrium constants (shown as the letter K) mean the reaction will go fairly far into completion, while low Ks mean the reaction will not go very far.

Before we calculate a K value for any chemical reaction, you need to know what equilibrium looks like. The reaction where you take N2O4 and turn it into NO2 or nitrous oxide will go to a certain level and then quit. The levels of each substance will remain the same as shown in this image:

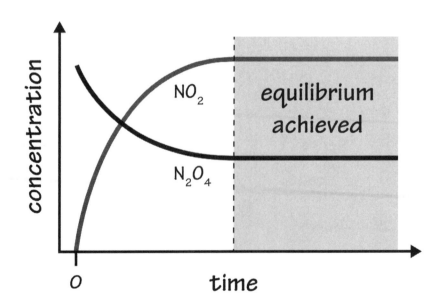

The reaction in this image does not go to completion at all, so the K value will be in the middle range of K values. This will be a reversible reaction as well because even at equilibrium, some N2O4 will transform into NO2 and vice versa, but the concentration will stay the same during the equilibrium phase. It's called dynamic equilibrium because it isn't as though nothing at all is happening.

Here's how you calculate the K for a chemical reaction. A common way to do this is to figure out the concentration of each substance in the reaction (reactants and products) at equilibrium. It does no good to do these things before equilibrium has been reached. An example is this reaction:

$$CO_2(g) + H_2(g) \rightleftharpoons CO(g) + H2O(g)$$

Now, measure the concentration of each gas in the reaction system and do this calculation:

$$K_c = \frac{[CO]\,[H_2O]}{[CO_2]\,[H_2]}$$

Essentially, these are the concentrations of the products multiplied together, then the concentration of the reactants multiplied together. You can imagine then that the higher the concentration of products, the greater the K will be. It will mean that the reaction is more likely to go to completion. *You need to write the equation in the number of moles of the product and reactants you have*.

You can sometimes guess at the K by knowing most of the concentrations of substances but not all. If you know all but one of them and the stoichiometry of the equation, you can determine the molar concentration of the one substance you don't know, and you then have your answer. There are also charts for equilibrium constants for specific reactions under defined conditions.

Let's Wrap This Up

Even if you don't remember the laws of thermodynamics, you should know what enthalpy and entropy mean. You should also remember that entropy will always increase unless energy is put into a chemical reaction (or any system in physics, nature, etc.). You should then know how this all works with chemical reactions, including whether or not a reaction will move spontaneously.

When you work with Gibbs free energy and change in enthalpy, you should know that a negative sign means the substances have less enthalpy in exothermic reactions because they give off heat (and have less innate heat of their own). Finally, understand that reactions in chemistry do not proceed to completion all the time; those that are reversible to some degree will have a K constant or *equilibrium constant* that will tell you to what degree a reaction goes to completion.

CHAPTER 11:

ELECTROCHEMISTRY

When you think of electricity, you probably don't think of chemistry but instead something related to physics. While physics courses cover electricity a great deal, a lot of electrical principles originate in chemistry. Electricity is the flow of electrons from one place to another. Most of the time, this flow of electrons is designed to do work of some kind, although you can imagine that lightning and static electricity in your living room carpet are less useful.

In this section, we will talk about some destructive electrochemical processes and those that are not nearly as destructive. Batteries, for example, are a perfect example of chemical electricity that does work. We will also talk about corrosion, which is a natural example of electrochemical changes seen every day.

Electrochemistry Basics

You cannot get far into studying electrochemistry without looking at the basic electrochemical cell. These cells have two electrodes sitting in an electrolyte solution. Electrons travel from one electrode to another through the solution. Two definitions you should know are these:

- **Anode**—the negatively-charged electrode that donates electrons in order to reduce another substance. It will release electrons into the electrolyte solution, where they travel to the cathode. The anode is what gets oxidized itself. (Remember how this works in redox reactions? It's the same thing happening over a longer distance.)
- **Cathode**—the positively-charged electrode that accepts electrons, getting oxidized as a result. When it does this, it will reduce the other substance in the anode.

In this process, the electrolyte solution is the medium that helps electrons travel from place to place. It is the solution highway where electrons go from anode to cathode. In almost all cases, the solvent is water, while the solute may be a salt, acid, or base. You need these solutes to have the ionic conduction necessary to have this process continue. The exception to the water-based system can be seen in batteries you use at home, which have solid electrolytes.

This is what an electrochemical system looks like:

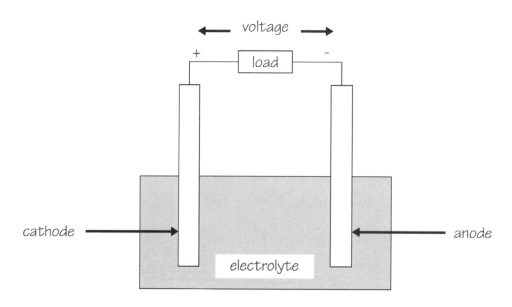

Components of a Cell

A good anode is one that is a strong reducing agent that conducts electricity well. It should be stable in water, low cost, and easily made. Common anode materials are lithium and zinc. A good cathode is an oxidizing agent that is also stable in the electrolyte solution. It should also be inexpensive and easy to make because it will get damaged in some way as part of the cell's processes.

You do need a good electrolyte as well—one that has good ionic conductivity but that won't interact with the electrodes in ways that will innately destroy them. It should be safe and must resist temperature fluctuations. Many alkali, salt, and acidic solutions will do this well.

Electrolysis

Galvanic cells are situations where chemical potential energy becomes electrical energy. On the other hand, electrolytic cells involve electrical energy that drives chemical reactions that would not otherwise happen without the addition of electricity. *This process is called electrolysis.*

Let's look at how electrolytic cells are supposed to work:

Suppose you take melted or molten sodium chloride, where the ions are freely moving to and from the different electrodes. This is the process used to make sodium metal and chlorine gas. The sodium metal is at the cathode, while the chlorine is at the anode. This will require a battery to add electrons to the system, but, if it works as predicted, it looks like this:

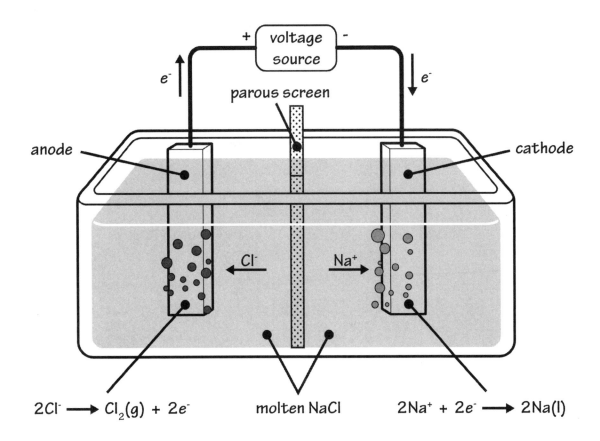

Do you see how the sodium chloride provides the ions to make chlorine gas and sodium metal, simply by adding or subtracting electrons to the different ions? Rather than electrons traveling from place to place, it's the ions themselves that move and that will either settle on the cathode or bubble off the anode. Note that this is not aqueous sodium chloride but molten salt; this is because sodium metal made in a watery environment would react and explode.

What happens with electrolysis of water? It turns out you can create hydrogen gas and oxygen gas by splitting water this way. You need to add sulfuric acid to the water so there will be extra hydrogen ions in the solution. The anode has oxygen, and the cathode has hydrogen gas. You basically have an oddly shaped system where you can bubble off the gases separately like this:

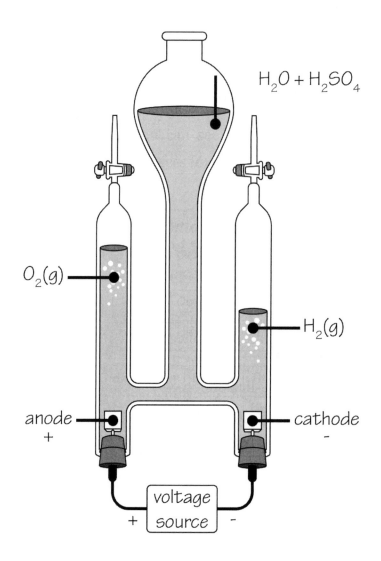

As you can see, this process does not happen by itself but happens best when you apply an energy source in the form of a battery of some kind.

Electroplating

You can see how electroplating would involve electrochemistry, with the goal of coating an object so it is more appealing or corrosion-resistant. Cadmium, gold, copper, silver, chromium, and tin are all able to be electroplated in some way. Jewelry, silverware, and tableware, as well as some industrial products, are electroplated for different reasons. The image for silver-plating a spoon is this one:

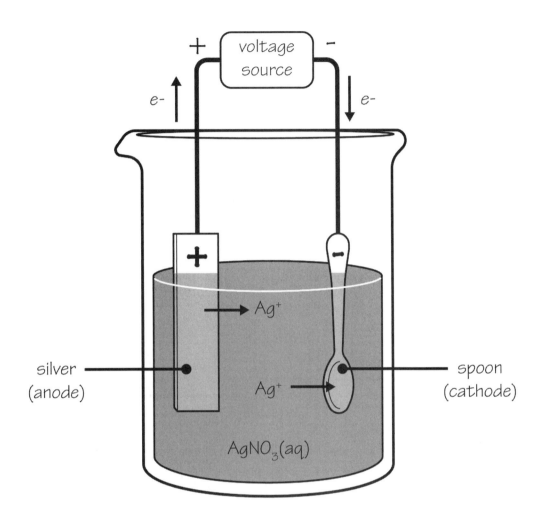

There is a silver anode which silver comes from. Silver nitrate is the ion in the solution. The cathode is the spoon which picks up the silver and gets coated. You would do this until you got a thickness you want; then you would be done.

Galvanic Cells

Galvanic cells are also called voltaic cells. These are specialized electrochemical cells that involve spontaneous redox reactions. Because these are spontaneous, you can produce electrical energy. You should separate the reduction and oxidation reactions when you write them, even when they do not operate that way.

One example of this is using a copper strip placed inside a silver nitrate solution. Copper in this solution will begin the immediate formation of silver metal and copper ions. The solution turns blue because copper ions are blue. The two half-reactions are these:

1. Oxidation: $Cu(s) \rightarrow Cu\ 2+$ (aq) and 2 electrons
2. Reduction: $2Ag+$ and 2 electrons $\rightarrow 2Ag$ (s)

These are put together to make an entire redox reaction in a single galvanic cell. NOTE: It takes two rounds of silver to make one round of copper in order to have a balanced equation.

The trick with galvanic cells is that they are spontaneous and do not require any specific voltage applied to the reaction. The oxidizing site is always the anode, while the reducing site is always the cathode. In this case, if you want the reaction to go to near completion, you need to put in twice as many moles of silver as you do copper. A salt bridge is used to close the circuit rather than any electrical wires. Often the salt bridge isn't part of the reaction per se but just carries current. The idea is to keep everything electrically neutral. It can look like this:

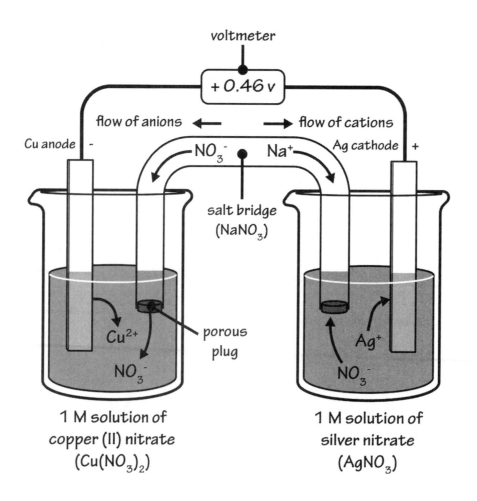

The salt bridge between the beakers is very necessary for electrical neutrality. There is a measurement called the cell potential, that takes into account the different electrical potentials existing in the two chambers. In the above example, there is a +0.46 volt difference between the two beakers.

Batteries

Batteries go one step further in what other electrochemical cells can do. These use electrochemical properties in order to make electrical currents that do work. You can imagine that galvanic cells do work to some degree because of the cell potential between them but are able to use this potential to do work by putting something that needs electricity into the surface.

Batteries can be single electrochemical cells or several of them. There is no such thing as an ideal battery that resists the elements, never runs out of power, or keeps the same voltage. The perfect battery for any job is the right size for its job, is inexpensive, and lasts as long as is reasonable for what you want to use it for.

You should know that there are two kinds of batteries; some are primary batteries and others are secondary batteries. We will talk about how these batteries operate soon. All batteries will generate some sort of electricity.

Primary Batteries

Primary batteries are single-use batteries. You know all about these. These are those you use and then throw away. The dry-cell battery is one of these. It is a zinc and carbon battery, where zinc is the anode and carbon is the cathode. The carbon is just a rod that is immersed in a manganese (IV) oxide paste that also contains zinc chloride, carbon powder, and a few other things. Zinc becomes a zinc ion, while several reactions happen at the cathode to create electrical energy. There is no salt bridge because you want to create an electrical potential you can use to make things work.

This is the inside of this type of battery:

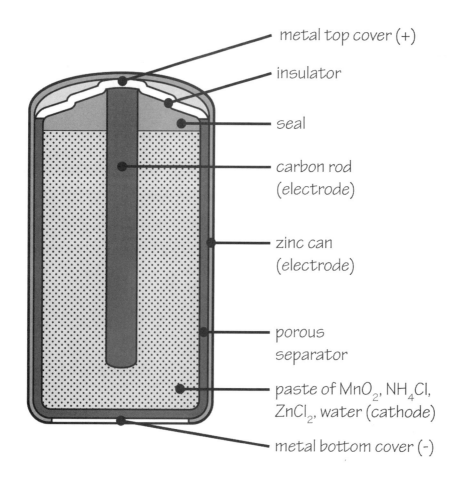

metal top cover (+)

insulator

seal

carbon rod
(electrode)

zinc can
(electrode)

porous
separator

paste of MnO_2, NH_4Cl,
$ZnCl_2$, water (cathode)

metal bottom cover (-)

Did you know? *All batteries you use (AAA, AA, C, and D) all carry the same voltage. The difference between these kinds of batteries is in the number of moles of electrons the battery can deliver. You can imagine that once the zinc runs out of these batteries, the battery will be "dead," and you will have to replace it. Also, the zinc ions leak out, which is why you shouldn't keep a battery in a device you aren't using repeatedly.*

Alkaline batteries can be used in place of the older zinc-carbon dry cell batteries; they are designed to eliminate some of the older cell's problems. The electrolytes here are alkaline—usually potassium hydroxide. Zinc solid is still used as the anode and becomes Zn2+ in the reaction. The cathode involves manganese dioxide (MnO2) which is also a solid.

Alkaline batteries are more energetic at three to five times that of the older batteries. Unfortunately, these can leak caustic potassium hydroxide, so they should also be removed from devices you are not immediately using. Some but not all of these are rechargeable. Never try to recharge those that aren't specifically rechargeable—they can expand and explode on you! This is what they look like:

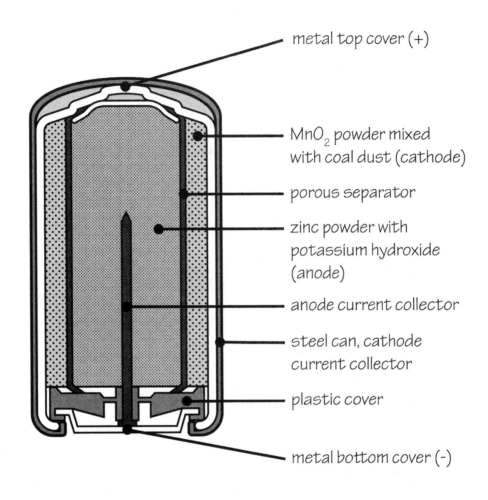

metal top cover (+)

MnO_2 powder mixed with coal dust (cathode)

porous separator

zinc powder with potassium hydroxide (anode)

anode current collector

steel can, cathode current collector

plastic cover

metal bottom cover (-)

Secondary Batteries

Secondary batteries are the only ones that are consistently rechargeable. These are your car batteries, smartphone batteries, and computer/tablet batteries. They are also called nickel-cadmium batteries. The cathode is coated with nickel, and the anode is coated with cadmium.

These are separated by sheeting and rolled up like a jelly-roll.

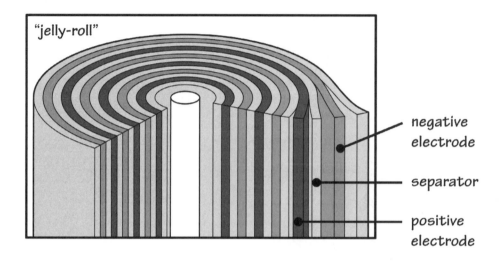

In these batteries, the cadmium becomes Cd2+ at the anode, while nickel dioxide solid (NiO2) at the anode becomes nickel hydroxide. The reactions put together look like this:

Reaction	Voltage
$Cd + 2OH^- \longrightarrow Cd(OH)_2 + 2e^-$	0.81 (cathode)
$NiO_2 + 2H_2O + 2e^- \longrightarrow Ni(OH)_2 + 2OH^-$	0.49 (anode)
$Cd + NiO_2 + 2H_2O \longrightarrow Cd(OH)_2 + Ni(OH)_2$	1.30 (combined)

Lithium-ion batteries are another type of secondary battery. These are rechargeable and are used in portable electronic devices. The battery looks like this:

Lithium-Ion Battery

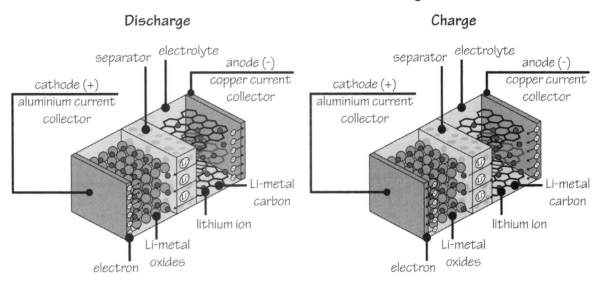

Fuel Cells

Fuel cells also convert chemical energy into electrical energy. They are like batteries in that way but need to be replenished with fuel in order to operate. Hydrogen is the most common fuel source for this sort of thing. These are used in satellite systems, boats, submarines, and some cars. Hydrogen and oxygen go into the fuel cell and generate power, giving off water as a waste product.

This is how they produce energy:

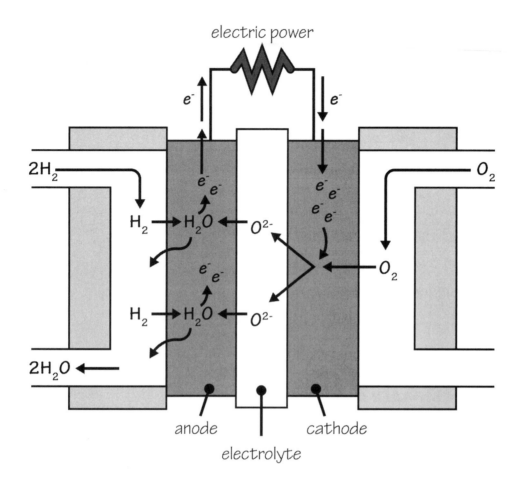

These types of fuel cells generate about 0.9 volts of electricity and are more efficient than batteries. They are expensive and tend to fail fairly easily, so don't expect them in too many devices you use every day.

Corrosion

If you look at any bridge that has been around for a while (or even the bumper of an old car), you will see evidence of corrosion at work. Corrosion happens to some but not all metals. Classical corrosion only happens to iron and things that contain iron; however, other metals will react with air to have some degree of tarnishing or destruction in the face of oxygen.

Highly reactive metallic elements like magnesium, zinc, tin, and aluminum are prone to some degree of corrosion, while copper and silver will tarnish easily. Each of these processes happens because the metal comes in contact with oxygen, undergoing an oxidative process to leave behind an iron oxide—which we call rust.

Corrosion is actually an electrochemical process. It results in the degradation of the metal and a rusty to greenish color on the metal's surface, depending on the metal involved. One famous example of corrosion is the Statue of Liberty. It came to the US as brown in color but oxidized over time to have its blue-green color as it is now. The reaction takes Cu metal and oxygen, resulting in Cu2O or copper (I) oxide. This is red in color. Over time, you get copper (II) oxide, which is black. These react with carbon dioxide to make copper carbonate, which is green.

Rust is another great example of corrosion. It requires iron, oxygen, and water. It does not take long for iron to oxidize in the presence of air. Iron will become iron (II) and will give off electrons that reduce oxygen under acidic conditions. This process then turns the oxygen atoms into water. Rust is actually iron (III) oxide, which is one step further from iron (III) oxide in the oxidation process.

While the Statue of Liberty is well-protected by its patina (it forms a layer that prevents deeper corrosion), this isn't the case with iron. Rust just flakes off, exposing more iron to get rusty as well. This figure shows you how this becomes an electrochemical process rather than just a chemical process:

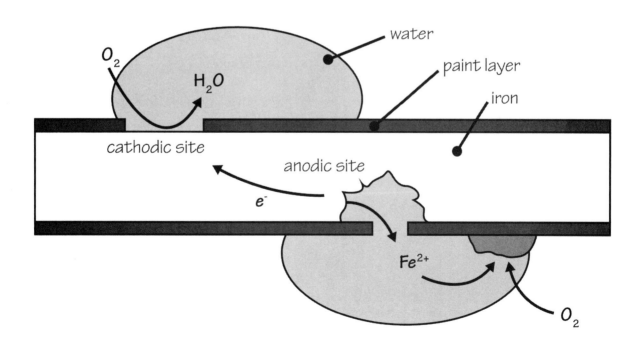

When it comes to the rusting of cars, electrolytes that conduct electricity speed the process up, so all the salt they put on icy, wet roads really increases the chance of rusting. Paint will prevent rusting from occurring, as you might imagine.

Other things to prevent rust include mixing iron with non-rusting metals. Stainless steel, for example, is iron mixed with a bit of chromium. Chromium does form an oxide layer on the surface of the steel, but it is protective against other rusting deeper into the object.

Galvanized steel or galvanized iron uses zinc to plate the iron. The idea behind this is that zinc will be more reactive than iron and will oxidize first. What this does is provide a zinc oxide coating on the steel object which protects the steel underneath.

You can do some really interesting stuff here to protect metals that are hard to coat or paint. You simply create a galvanic cell situation in which you make the metal you want to protect the cathode. Consider an underground iron storage tank that you want to keep from rusting. What you would do is to connect it to a zinc or magnesium metal object; this will be called the sacrificial anode. The anode gets oxidized instead of the holding tank by being the anode. The anode gets replaced periodically to keep the cathode tank more pristine.

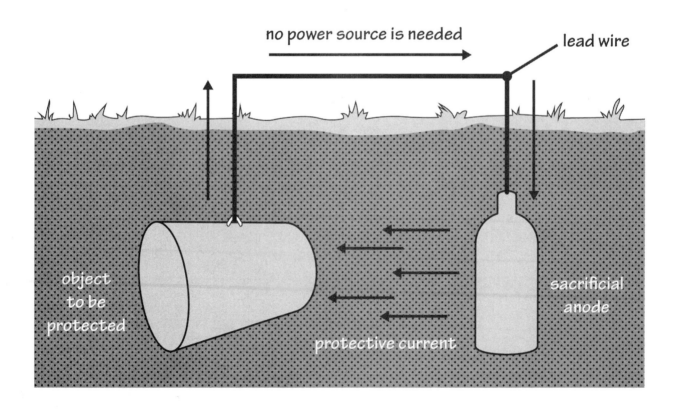

Let's Wrap This Up

Who knew that a few electrons would amount to real energy you can use? It turns out that these redox reactions are able to do a great deal to generate useable energy. The fuel cell and batteries are both systems where chemistry is recruited to help create the energy you are able to use and sometimes recharge afterward.

Corrosion and rust are another thing altogether. These oxidation reactions tend to destroy important metallic objects unless the corrosion creates a protective layer around the metallic object (as you'll see at the Statue of Liberty, for example).

SECTION 6:

GASES, LIQUIDS, AND SOLIDS

This section is devoted to studying the properties of liquids, solids, and gases. Gases are interesting in the way they mix. The ideal gas laws help us determine how an *ideal* gas should behave. Some gases behave *close enough* to ideal gases to use the ideal gas laws in your calculations, while others will not. Liquids and solids also have unique properties as well; once you know these, you will be able to understand what makes each substance different from the next.

CHAPTER 12:

GASES

Now that you know the different states of matter and a bit more about bonding and intermolecular forces, it's time to dig deeper into how the different states of matter behave. We will start with gases, which may or may not have forces existing between the molecules. As you will see, gases are far more *empty space* than they are actual molecules. For this reason, the forces between these molecules are minimal.

Gases are lightweight compared to the same volume of solid or liquid. What do we mean when we say this? In order words, which weighs more, a kilogram of air or a kilogram of solid lead? This is a trick question because they have exactly the same mass (one kilogram). What you really want to know is what volume does a kilogram of each substance take up? This gives you an idea of the density of each substance.

A kilogram of air takes up about 0.77 cubic meters (think of a cube with sides equal to 1 meter each). Lead is much denser than air, with a density of 11.342 kilograms per cubic meter, so one kilogram is just 0.088 cubic meters.

This is also a trick question because it doesn't state the conditions. You need to know the conditions in wgich you are doing the experiment, especially when it comes to air (or any gas). Most of the time, if conditions are not listed, you can assume *standard conditions*, which are set conditions of standard temperature and pressure.

Standard conditions: You call this *STP*, meaning *Standard Temperature and Pressure*. In IUPAC terms, these conditions are 0 degrees Celsius and 105 pascals. If you used Imperial units, this would instead be 60 degrees Fahrenheit and one atmosphere.

Why would this make any difference? It wouldn't make a gigantic distance with solid lead, but the difference with air would be remarkable. As you will see, the density of a gas or the volume it occupies is greatly dependent on its temperature and pressure. Gases are incredibly compressible, so the same kilogram of air at 1 atmosphere takes up much more space than the same kilogram of air under higher pressures (when you put the squeeze on the gas molecules). The ideal gas laws help explain why this is the case.

Kinetic Theory and the Study of Gases

When you study the kinetic theory of gases, what you are really looking at is the movement of gas molecules. Kinetics is the study of movement in general. Gaseous molecules are very free to move randomly within whatever physical space they are in. Heat energy or temperature determines how much kinetic energy or movement they have. You can use these tiny bits of molecular kinetic energy in order to see what the observable aspects of gases look like.

The pressure of any gas inside a container is a function of how much movement they have in the physical space they are in. High pressure in a gas could mean a few molecules with a lot of kinetic energy or a lot of molecules with less kinetic energy. It would be like measuring how often people bumped into one another in a subway station. If there is a lot of movement, people will collide, even if they aren't too close together. If they are crowded in the station already, it doesn't take a lot of individual movement to get plenty of collisions.

When you study the kinetics of gases, you need to take these things into account:

- ✓ Gases are made up of much more dead space than they are of actual molecules. In fact, the space taken up by the molecules themselves doesn't even count in the ideal gas calculations.
- ✓ Molecules of gas don't attract or repel each other, and they don't attract or repel the walls of the container.
- ✓ The molecules move completely randomly and never lose kinetic energy when they bounce off from one another. This means we do not see them as sticky. They really do bounce without losing their energy.
- ✓ Temperature and kinetic energy are directly proportional to one another. It's the average kinetic energy of all the molecules you need to consider here, even if they don't all move at the same rate.

The average gas molecule under STP conditions moves at between 0.1 and 1 kilometer per second and bumps into about 10,000,000,000 other molecules during a single second. As the temperature increases, the kinetic energy of the gas will proportionately increase. Kinetic energy theory helps to describe the behavior we see in the different ideal gas laws we will talk about in a minute.

What are Ideal and Non-Ideal Gases?

An ideal gas is a lot like other ideal things. It is theoretical and doesn't really exist in real life. An ideal gas doesn't have any interactions between the gas molecules. This makes it simpler than it otherwise would be to explain the gas's properties with a lot of different interactions happening in the substance.

Some gases are not ideal but are considered close enough because they have what are called elastic conditions when they bump into one another. This means they may bump into one another, but neither sticks to another. Chemists call these *point-like collisions*. Other ideal gas situations include the fact that the gas molecules should be singular, or a *monatomic gas*. Some diatomic gases like oxygen and nitrogen are small enough and behave in ways enough like the monatomic gases to be counted as such.

Air mixtures and carbon dioxide gases are heavy but also behave a lot like ideal gases under most conditions. The higher the temperature and the lower the pressure of a gaseous system, the more likely it will behave *ideally*. This is because the kinetic energy or molecular speed and activity overcome any interactions between the molecules. Lower pressures also mean that gas molecules have fewer neighbors to bump into.

Did you know? Gas molecules in our atmosphere are super-hot high in the thermosphere around the earth (between 85 and 600 kilometers above the earth). Temperatures reach 2000 degrees Celsius. If you were up that high, however, you might feel okay or even cool. Why is this? Even though the molecules are moving about wildly because of the high temperatures involved, there are so few of these in the atmosphere that high up that they rarely touch your skin. Because of this low air density, you just don't feel the heat behind these energetic molecules.

According to the rules around ideal gases, one mole of any ideal gas takes up about 22.7 liters of space, as long as the conditions are *standard* (0 degrees Celsius and 105 pascals of pressure). These are the IUPAC standard conditions.

Gases behaving less ideal are these:

- ✓ Those with strong intermolecular forces (like water vapor)
- ✓ Those at lower temperatures
- ✓ Those at higher pressures
- ✓ Very heavy gases

There is a term called the compressibility factor Z, which doesn't make much sense, as it has no dimensions. It is a number that describes how much a given gas is deviating from an ideal gas in terms of its behavior.

There are a number of interrelated laws used to describe ways that ideal gases behave. Each of them looks at just one aspect of gas behavior; however, *real* ideal gases behave according to each of these gas laws together. Let's look at these laws:

Boyle's Gas Law

This law assumes that the mass of the gas and its temperature are held constant. It helps describe the relationship between the volume of a gas and its pressure. This one is easy to understand. If you decrease the volume, or *space*, for a gas, you essentially compress it, increasing the pressure in the shrinking container.

Robert Boye described it using this equation:

$$Pressure = K(1/volume)$$

In this case, the term K is a proportionality constant. Does the constant K have a value of any kind? Not really. All you can say is that if you multiply the pressure and volume of a gaseous system, you get a constant number.

Charles's Law

Jacques Charles developed his law of gases about a century after Boyle did (in 1878). Charles's law is similar, except that the pressure and mass are kept the same. He was able to determine that the temperature and volume of any gas are proportional to one another. The idea behind this is that if you take a hot-air balloon, for example, and warm up the gas you put into it, the balloon will expand proportionally to the temperature of the gas.

Charles was able to determine specifically that each degree Celsius you add to the system means you will gain about 1/273.15 times the original volume. If the volume at 0 degrees Celsius is called Vo and you try to reach another volume (say Vt, where t is the added temperature), you get this equation:

$$Vt = V0(273.15 + {}^t/273.15)$$

The other way to look at this is like this: $\frac{Vt}{V0} = \frac{Tt}{T0}$

Just as in Boyle's Law, you would get the fact that the volume equals some constant multiplied by the temperature. Again, there isn't a consistent value of this constant; it depends on the system.

Gay-Lussac's Law

Gay-Lussac's law is another ideal gas law. If you have figured out the trend, you can see where a comparison hasn't yet been made between the temperature and pressure of an ideal gas system. Guy Lussac observed in 1802 that if you kept the mass and volume the same but changed the temperature and pressure, you would see that the temperature and pressure are directly proportional to one another. This means that dividing pressure and temperature gives rise to yet another proportionality constant.

Avogadro's Law

These ideal gas laws bring us back to Amedeo Avogadro, who determined that if you took a specific volume of gaseous molecules at a constant temperature and pressure and counted every molecule (something not recommended, by the way), you would get the same number of molecules in that volume, regardless of the identity of the gas. This means that volume and the number of molecules are equally proportional to one another. One mole of any gas contains exactly the same number of molecules as Avogadro's number (6.022 x 10^{23}). Every single mole of any gas at STP values has the same volume.

Putting it All Together

You can finally put this collection of gas laws into one law that incorporates real numbers you can measure by using what's called the *ideal gas law*. You need to know at least some of the three state variables we've been talking about. These are Pressure, Volume, and Absolute Temperature. The law essentially means this:

$$PV = nRT = NkT$$

The initials stand for these things:

- ✓ n = the number of moles in the system
- ✓ R = the universal gas constant, which is 8.3145 Joules/mole Kelvin
- ✓ N = the number of molecules
- ✓ k = Boltzmann constant, which is 1.38066 x 10^{-23} Joules/degrees Kelvin
- ✓ k = R/NA where NA is Avogadro's number

If you decide to use standard (STP) conditions, you would be able to figure out that one mole of any ideal gas would take up about 22.4 liters.

Let's Wrap This Up

- ✓ Gas laws are made for ideal gases, even though there is no such thing as an ideal gas in real life.
- ✓ Many gases will behave close enough to real gases to make gas laws helpful in understanding them.
- ✓ Gases tend to be much more empty space than actual molecules. The space taken up by the molecules is negligible compared to the empty space between them.
- ✓ Temperature, pressure, and volume are all related to one another when it comes to gases.
- ✓ Gas molecules have kinetic energy based on their temperature. Thermal energy gets translated into movement, or *kinetic energy.*
- ✓ An ideal gas under STP conditions takes up 22.4 liters of space.

CHAPTER 13:

LIQUIDS AND SOLIDS

Solids and liquids are more interesting from an intramolecular forces perspective, mostly because the molecules are closer to one another and sluggish enough to have time to interact with one another. As you can imagine, these interactions are not the same from substance to substance. Water molecules interact far more differently than molecules of methane liquid, for example. We've studied some aspects of liquids and intermolecular forces already.

In this chapter, we talk more about how these forces shape the properties of each type of liquid or solid substance. Solids and liquids carry unique properties that depend on what happens to the substances on a molecular level. You will hopefully learn why honey flows with increased viscosity, but that gasoline has much less viscosity than most other substances in nature.

As you probably already know, not all liquids are created the same. Some seem to like each other and mix well together, but if you've ever studied your salad dressing, you know that if you set it out for long, the oil will settle on top, and the watery parts will stay on the bottom. Your glass of milk seems consistent from top to bottom, but if you leave it out too long, a watery layer separates from a clot that doesn't seem at all to be dissolved in the watery part.

Most of the chemistry of liquids involves solutions. These are situations where there is a solvent and some type of completely inseparable solute dissolved in it. This is the kind of situation you see with most salts. Your milk, on the other hand, is a colloid. These are deceiving because they look as though all the parts are together, but in reality, the white part of milk is butterfat in globules that are just suspended in the watery part. Given enough time, the layers will separate out. We will talk about colloids later.

As you know, liquids have the ability to flow. This is because their intermolecular forces (the forces between the different molecules) are weak enough to allow the different molecules to move. They are not fixed when it comes to their position relative to other molecules. Unlike intramolecular forces, the atoms in the molecules can shift rapidly as they tumble around, which accounts for the *fluidity* of these substances.

Solid substances have much stronger intermolecular or intramolecular forces that do not allow for much, if any, movement within the substance. All molecules vibrate to some degree, but in solids, this is about all the movement they can get. If you try to compress a real solid, you will not be able to do it very much. This is also true of liquids, even though they flow from a molecular level.

Intermolecular Forces in Liquids

The forces between liquids can be repulsive or attractive. Just like magnets are attracted, if you touch the negative pole with the positive one, you will get the attraction of molecules when a polar molecule has its negative end in close contact with the positive end of another molecule that is also polar. Because these molecules are constantly moving, you can imagine that, in the shuffle, there will be times when you don't get attraction; instead, the molecules are repulsive to one another. If this happens, it is temporary because, in the next moment, the molecules will shift until they are more *comfortable* with one another or are in a better position to attract one another.

Nonpolar substances like many organic molecules (think gasoline) do not have polarity. Without this polarity, these molecules do not have many attractive forces between them. This is why they tend to be thinner and boil at lower temperatures than liquids with polar molecules in them.

So, when we talk about intermolecular forces, we mean things like hydrogen bonding and London dispersion forces. You already know about these forces and how they are not truly bonds but are essentially attractive forces that allow for attraction between molecules just as much as they do within molecules.

There are many properties of liquids that you have most likely observed but didn't realize were from specific intramolecular interactions. Let's look at these unique properties of liquids:

Cohesion

The property of cohesion could be considered the opposite of slipperiness. Liquids you see as slippery have very little cohesion. An example of this would be any type of oil. You use oil to keep things from sticking together. Cohesion on a molecular level means that the molecules have high levels of interaction with one another, while low cohesion equates to low levels of interaction with one another.

Organic molecules with only carbon and hydrogen in them do not participate much in the known intermolecular forces like hydrogen bonding or van der Waals forces. They do have London dispersion forces, which are the weakest type of intermolecular *bonding*. This lack of sticky interaction with one another means the liquid made from these molecules will be slippery rather than sticky.

Water, by comparison, is very sticky. Think of a drop of water that sticks to a surface and doesn't spread out nicely. This drop of water is able to stay nice and elevated on a leaf when you see dew in the morning because of the hydrogen bonding between water molecules. You will see that water has a lot of properties like high cohesion that you wouldn't expect to see out of such a small molecule.

Cohesion is strongly related to surface tension. You've seen surface tension in action if you have ever seen an insect walk swiftly upon the water, even if it is clearly liquid water. Water has a high surface tension, meaning it takes a greater deal of force before you can break the *tension* of the surface created between the liquid and the gas (*air* in most cases) above it. If the same insect tried to walk on a liquid made of an organic molecule like benzene or gasoline, it would have a much harder time doing this. It is the surface tension that makes the water droplet round.

Let's talk about adhesion, which is similar in some ways to the cohesive properties of a liquid. This image describes the difference between these two properties of liquids:

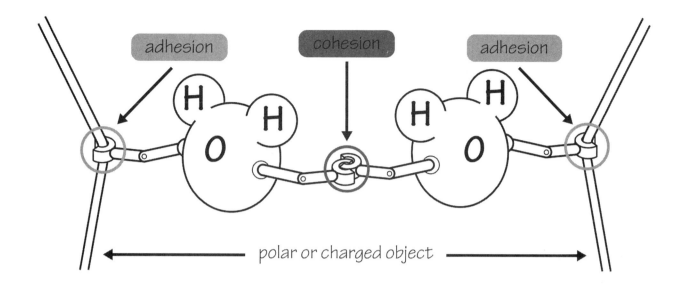

adhesion   cohesion   adhesion

polar or charged object

Adhesion

Adhesion is similar to cohesion but involves attractive forces between two dissimilar molecules. When you see a dewdrop hanging off a leaf, it is adhesion that keeps the droplet attached to the leaf itself. Adhesion helps a liquid stick (or not) to the container it is in and to any other liquids near it. Water has a meniscus in a test tube or other narrow tube because its adhesion to the tube itself is great enough to overcome the effects of gravity. You will not see the same meniscus if you put a nonpolar organic liquid in the same test tube. This is what a meniscus looks like:

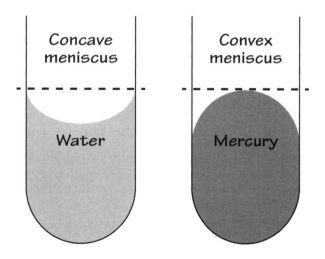

Concave meniscus — Water

Convex meniscus — Mercury

Water has a concave meniscus because adhesion is a stronger force than cohesion, so the molecules of water prefer to stick to the test tube. The water looks like it is creeping up the test tube sides. If the liquid is mercury, you will have a convex meniscus. This is because this substance has more cohesion between the mercury molecules than it does adhesion. At the edges of the test tube, the mercury will not stick very well.

Capillary action is also related to adhesive forces. When you narrow the tube, you have a greater number of molecules next to the tube compared to those next to each other. This translates to a greater overall adhesive force with respect to the tube that can overcome the effects of gravity and the adhesive forces between the water molecules themselves. This figure shows how narrower tubes have a greater capillary action:

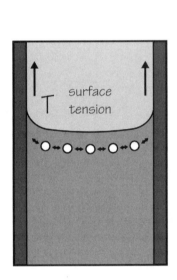 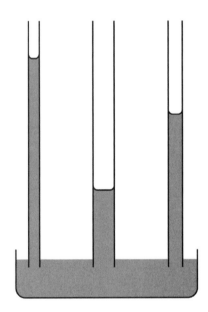

Viscosity

You have seen viscosity in action whenever you try to pour something like honey or motor oil from a container. These liquids are very slow-moving. This resistance to flowing movement is referred to as viscosity. Water is much less viscous than oil, as you can easily demonstrate when trying to pour them.

In general, you will see less viscosity in liquids made from smaller molecules and in those where the London dispersion forces are weak. Pentane is a five-carbon hydrocarbon with even less viscosity than water, even though it is bigger. The lack of strong forces between the molecules increases the slipperiness or movement of molecules past each other. When you pour it, it will pour easily.

With viscosity, size matters a great deal. A large hydrocarbon does not have a lot of polarity or intermolecular bonding happening, but because it is large, the molecules just don't slide past one another well. Motor oil, for example, is made from large and easily bendable carbon-containing molecules. Getting them to slide past one another would be like having to untangle a bowl of spaghetti noodles so they could individually slide out of a bowl.

The temperature has a great deal to do with how viscous something is. In your car, for example, the thick oil you put in will be a great deal thinner and more lubricating once it is in the inner workings of your warm vehicle. If it happens to be -40 degrees Fahrenheit outside when you start your car, not so much. Temperature adds kinetic energy to the molecules, which allows even larger molecules to disentangle themselves more easily in the liquid soup where they reside. The liquid itself then will be less viscous.

Complex Liquids Made from More than One Molecule Type

Most liquids are not just made of a single molecule but are instead combinations of more than one molecule. Water is just H2O molecules together, but if you are dealing with anything in it (like salt or sugar), you are talking about a _solution_ rather than just water, which is the solvent. You know that salt and sugar can be solutes, but things like gaseous carbon dioxide (CO2) and other liquids (like ethanol) can also serve as solutes.

You know already that _like dissolves like_, which means that polar solvents like polar solutes and nonpolar solvents like nonpolar solutes. This explains why you use turpentine for cleaning up after using oil paint and water to clean up after using acrylic paints.

There are other liquids besides solutions, as we've mentioned. Emulsions, suspensions, and colloids are all types of liquids that do not involve any type of dissolving of one substance into another. Emulsions happen when you mix any two liquids that wouldn't normally mix with one another. Your mayonnaise is an emulsion containing vinegar, egg yolks, and oil (with or without lemon juice). You just need to combine them vigorously to get your emulsion. This figure shows an oil in water and a water in oil emulsion:

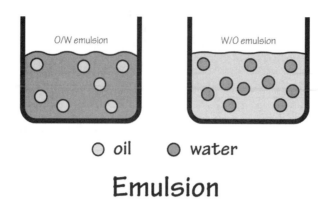

O oil ● water

Emulsion

Both colloids and suspensions are made from particles that wouldn't normally dissolve in the liquid mixing with the liquid in some way that doesn't allow for their separation easily. Colloids have such tiny particles that separation will not happen, while suspensions have larger particles that are heavy enough to separate relatively easily. This image is one that shows the size difference in solutes necessary to determine what type of liquid substance about which you are talking:

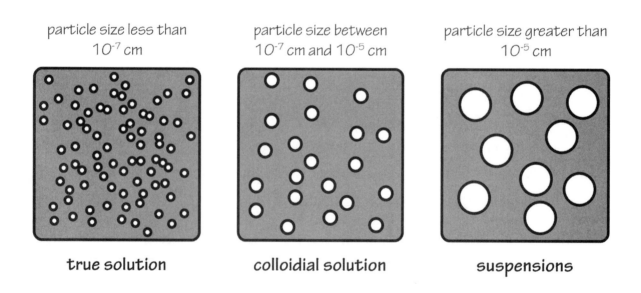

There are other phase-related mixtures you may not have thought of as being suspensions or colloids. You can see these are everyday things with which you come into contact that involve just about any combination of phases mixed together:

Simple Colloid Mixture Examples

Colloid Type	Mixture	Examples
aerosols	liquid particles • gas medium	mist, fog, hairspray
solid aerosols	solid particles • gas medium	smoke, dust, volcanic ash
fooms	gas particles • liquid medium	whipped cream, bubble bath, fire retardant
solid fooms	gas particles • solid medium	inoculation foam, yoga mats, memory foam
emulsions	liquid particles • liquid medium	mayonnaise, milk, salad dressing
sols	solid particles • liquid medium	blood, paint, mud
solid sols	solid particles • solid medium	gemstones, colored glass
gels	liquid particles • solid medium	cheese, jam, rubber

Milk is interesting. If you buy fresh milk, you are getting a true suspension. Before too long, it will separate its components. The milk you buy at a store is usually a colloid. It is *homogenized*, meaning that the fat globules are so tiny, they do not separate.

Characteristics of Solids

Some solids look so similar to the naked eye, you can't tell them apart. Table sugar and table salt look very similar, except when you look very closely at their crystals. That's one of the unique aspects of crystals. They have a very unique crystalline shape based entirely on their molecular structure and how the molecules interact with one another in solid form.

Salt is simple. It's sodium chloride in a square shape when in crystalline form. In the end, it looks a lot like this:

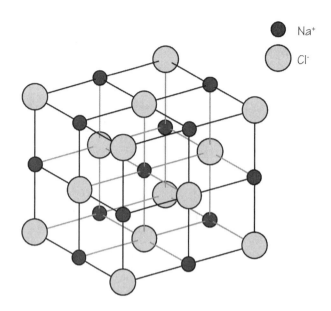

Na$^+$

Cl$^-$

Sugar is more complex and forms more interesting shapes as the complicated molecules find ways of interacting with each other that don't involve a lot of movement between the molecules. X-ray crystallography can be used to see what these interesting lattices look like.

Most liquid substances are denser when they become solids. The molecules condense into tight places where the energy necessary to keep the molecules together is in a low. Ice or solid water is a major exception. You can easily see why when you look at ice from a molecular standpoint.

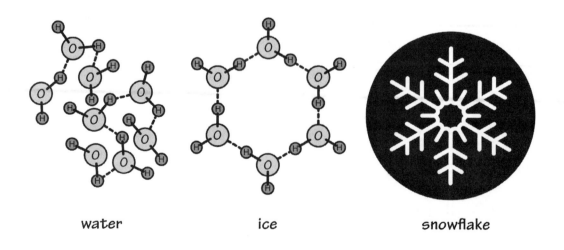

water   ice   snowflake

Now you can finally see why ice is so lightweight (less dense) than liquid water AND why snowflakes are naturally hexagonal. Cool, isn't it?

Solids can be crystalline or non-crystalline. You have seen crystals so far but you also need to think about other things—metals, wood, or window glass. The definition of a solid is anything that has a defined shape and size without needing any type of container to hold it. You can easily identify these things by their obvious immobility when you try to compress them.

Solids maintain their shape because they have strong attractive forces between the molecules or atoms involved that exceed the force needed to pull them apart. These are low-energy molecules that don't have enough of their own energy to be in any other position than the one they find themselves in when the solid forms.

Crystalline solids are well-organized in shapes specifically designed to fit their molecular shape. Non-crystals are also called an amorphous solid that are not necessarily precisely arranged. Glass is an amorphous solid with no particular order to its silicates within. If you make these same molecules behave in a crystalline way, you get something like quartz, which is a crystal made of silicates. The major difference between these two isn't the substances they are made from but in how they are made. These differences go on to cause one or the other type of solid.

Being a crystal means several things for a solid. It affects their density and the way they conduct electricity through them, for example. When you look specifically at crystalline solids, you will see that there are four different types of these:

- **Molecular solids** – made from any molecule that is itself held together by some type of strong covalent bond. Each molecule has its own structure, which can be large or small. It's these molecules that interact in specific ways with each other to make the solid.
- **Network solids** – there are no defined molecules in a network solid. Carbon is a classic example of this. In one arrangement of carbon, you have graphite, but in the other, you have diamonds. For sure, these look very different from one another, even though the atoms in them are the same. Atoms that are able to do this type of magic are said to have _allotropy_. This shows you why diamond and graphite look different from one another:

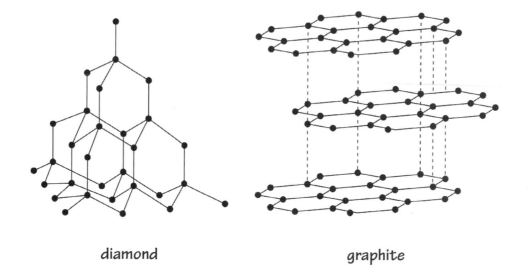

diamond   graphite

- **Ionic solids** – similar to network solids only in that there aren't any distinct molecules held by covalent bonding. There are instead clusters of molecules held by ionic bonding. You know these crystals well. These are all the different salt crystals you can imagine.
- **Metallic solids** – the common metals you know (silver, iron, lead, etc.). These are held through metallic bonding; metallic bonds allow for atoms within the solid to easily slide back and forth against each other (up to a point). We call that having *malleability*. Metallic solids will also conduct electricity as part of their main features.

Solids have unique properties too. These properties help define them and tell chemists what they are best used for. The properties are malleability, hardness, density, conductivity, and optical transmission.

Conductivity

Conductivity makes you think of electricity and wires, right? Well, inside most wires are things like copper, which conduct electricity very well. The reason they do this is because the atoms are a lot like atomic nuclei living in a soup of electrons. The atoms aren't too picky about which electrons they have and those they want to share. The electrons floating around in the outer shell of these atoms are free to travel; by doing so, they conduct electricity. Electricity is nothing more than floating electrons traveling from place to place. This image shows how the conductivity of electricity works in a metallic substance:

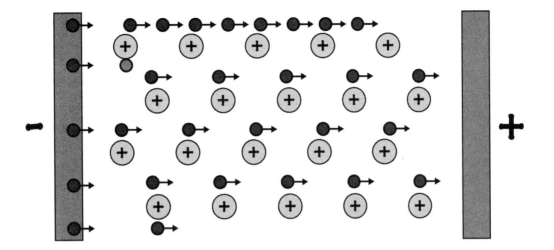

Anything that will not conduct electricity effectively is called an electrical insulator. It is an electrical insulator like rubber that you put around wires so you don't make direct contact with the electricity.

The thermal conductivity of metals is slightly different from electrical conductivity. Most metals that conduct electricity also conduct heat. You want all of your pots and pans to be made from metal so they can transfer the heat from your burner to your food effectively. Temperature is a reflection of the movement of molecules. You need to have molecular movement in order to have heat transferred through the solid substance. Solids that are too rigid internally will not conduct heat effectively, while those that are more movable internally will conduct heat.

Molecules and atoms that are metallic and conduct heat do not have movement in any specific direction. In other words, you will not get an atom of copper to move any great distance when you apply heat to it. But, you will get movement enough so the copper atom can bump against other copper atoms, generating heat. Again, if the solid is too rigid like you would see in a network solid, you don't get any thermal conductivity.

Graphite is interesting. It conducts both heat and electricity, even though it is not metallic. Researchers have made use of this by creating carbon nanotubes, which are essentially tubular graphite. These tubes conduct electricity and heat fairly well.

Malleability

Malleability and ductility are similar. You know something is malleable when you can take a hammer to it and bend it into a sheet, similar to sheet-metal. Metals are very malleable, which is something blacksmiths have used for millennia to make all sorts of things using heat and physical pressure out of blobs of metal. Metals are malleable because their atoms do not care very much about structure and do not take on any crystalline form. Ductility is the ability to take that same blob of metal and make a long wire out of it. Metalworkers know exactly how much pressure they need to apply and at what temperature it is necessary to get metal to bend or stretch.

Melting Point

You can get almost any metal to deform in some way simply by allowing it to melt. Like any solid characteristic, the melting point depends on the atomic and molecular structure of the solid. If there are strong bonds between the different molecules, it will take a lot of heat energy to melt them. Things like sugar can be melted easily because the bonds between the sugar molecules are weak. Stronger bonds happen in ionic solids, certain network solids, and metallic solids. The melting point of each substance depends on how strong the intermolecular forces are.

You know that some metals have lower melting points than others. Mercury is a metal that is liquid at room temperature. This means it has a very low boiling point. Others have a high melting point, such as tungsten, which melts at 3,422 degrees Celsius. Other solids have melting points too. Sodium chloride melts at 801 degrees Celsius, and a network solid like graphite melts at a whopping 4489 degrees Celsius. Ionic/salt bonds are weaker than most covalent or metallic bonds, which is reflected in their lower melting point.

Density

Density is the mass per any unit of volume. The density of any solid depends on how the different solid atoms or molecules are packed together. Metal atoms have irregular packing of atoms, and salts and other solids often have unique packing strategies that affect their overall density. Gold is packed in such a way as to be very dense. You already know that lead is dense but not as dense as gold (19.3 grams per cubic centimeter for gold versus 11.33 grams per cubic centimeter for lead).

The size of the molecules makes a difference. Large molecules cannot pack as closely together as small molecules. A jar with large jelly beans will have fewer beans than a jar packed with small jelly beans. If you have beans that are small AND large, you get an even greater density because the small beans can tuck into the spaces with the larger beans. Ionic solids are exactly like this, accounting for their high density. You already know that ice isn't particularly dense because of the geometry of its packed molecules. This image shows you why packing makes a difference in determining solid density.

Differences in Packing

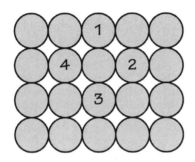 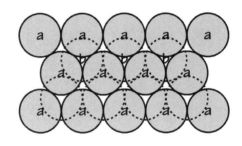

Let's Wrap This Up

Liquids and solids have unique properties you can identify by what's going on at a molecular level. Liquids tend to like other liquids similar to them. This means polar molecules like other polar molecules; they will dissolve into one another easily. Polar liquids like water will not mix well with nonpolar molecules like oil or gasoline. The properties of a liquid, such as the surface tension, viscosity, and others are related to the intermolecular forces between the liquid atoms and molecules.

Solids are crystalline, or amorphous. You learned about the different types of solids and their properties, such as their melting point, electrical conductivity, and malleability. Again, these properties can easily be explained when you know the chemistry of the different molecules and atoms involved in the solid.

SECTION 7:
ACID BASE CHEMISTRY

In this section, you will learn all about acids and bases. You probably know about things like battery acid, but the world of acids and bases is much broader than that. There are many different types of acids and bases (or alkalis) that interact with one another in fascinating ways. We will talk about what buffers are and when you would use them. Titrations are laboratory experiments at which we will also look more carefully.

CHAPTER 14:

ACIDS AND BASES

Before we get too far into what acids and bases are, you need to first look at what we really mean by *pH*. Then we will talk about acids and bases from a chemistry standpoint. It turns out that there are several definitions of what these mean. Let's dive in with the basics and go from there.

Acids, Bases, and pH

You can think of pH as being the *power of hydrogen* because it relates to the concentration of hydrogen in an aqueous solution. By *aqueous*, we mean *water*. You can technically use a pH scale outside of water, but when it comes to almost all situations, you need water.

You also need to remember that, while pH does relate to the concentration of hydrogen in water, there is no such thing as hydrogen ions floating around in water. Hydrogen doesn't do that; it needs a buddy of some kind to hang onto. In most cases, this buddy is a water molecule. In fact, water is always breaking down and building back up its physical H2O state—even when it is sitting by itself without any solute in it. The reaction it goes through is this:

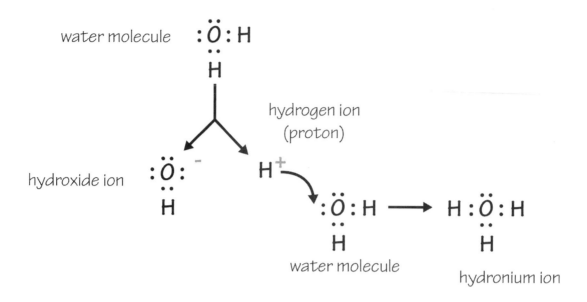

water molecule

hydrogen ion (proton)

hydroxide ion

water molecule

hydronium ion

What this means is that instead of measuring the hydrogen ion concentration, you are really looking at the hydronium ion concentration. Its opposite, the hydroxide ion, is just fine by itself. The truth is that neither stays by itself for long because the reverse reaction happens just as easily.

The pH is nothing but the negative base 10 logarithm of the hydronium ion in water. The scale goes from 0 to 14. Anything you measure that has a pH greater than 7 is basic, while anything you measure with a pH less than 7 is acidic. You need to know that this scale can be useless if you are dealing with very strong acids or bases. In such a case, it is possible to have a pH less than zero or greater than 14 (but it isn't common).

It is sometimes hard to figure out why a low number indicates more hydrogen ions (or acidity) and why a high number indicates low hydrogen ion concentrations. Let's work backward to determine why this would be.

Let's say you have two solutions. Solution A has a hydrogen ion concentration of 0.001 moles per liter, and the second one (solution B) has a hydrogen ion concentration of 0.00000001 M. Get out your math brain and figure out what the concentration is in when you use 10 to the power of something:

Solution A: 10^{-3} The log of this is -3, so the pH is 3 (acidic)

Solution B: 10^{-8} The log of this is -8, so the pH is 8 (basic)

It makes sense, right? Now you can see how this works. In plain water, the pH is 7, with a hydrogen ion concentration of 0.0000001. What is the hydroxide (OH-) concentration? It turns out that it is the same in plain water. If you wanted to look at what's called the pOH, you would calculate the log of the concentration of hydroxide ions and get the negative of the log to get a pOH of 7, as well. Add those two numbers up and you get 14. This is a nice trick because you can assume this fact:

The pH + the pOH = 14

Water: $H_2O \rightarrow H_3O+$ and OH-

The concentration of each is 10^{-7} or .0000001 moles per liter

One strange catch is that the pH depends on the temperature. The pH at *neutral* equals 7, which depends on the temperature of the solution to be 25 degrees Celsius, or about room temperature. Neutral pH is less than 7 if you bump up the temperature at all. Neutral pH is just 6.14 at the boiling point of water (100 degrees Celsius).

How do you measure the pH of something? There are several ways to do this. If you had a fancy setup with a calibrated electrode, it would be easy. The electrode could electrically check the hydronium ion concentration, and then you would have it. You can also use a pH indicator strip to rough out a reasonable number.

There is a universal pH indicator strip treated with chemicals that change color according to the pH. The colors on the strip are arranged in rainbow order, with red indicating a strong acid and purple or blue indicating a strong base. These work because the chemicals in the paper are color-changing according to the pH they are found in.

There will be a chart you can use to read it. It looks a lot like this:

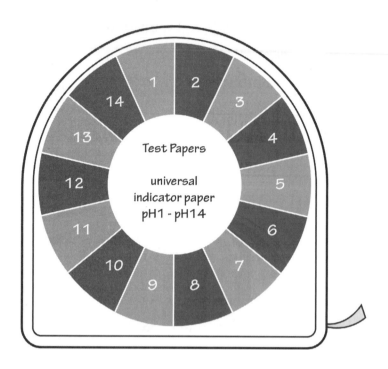

Litmus paper is much simpler. There are just two colors, with red being acidic and blue being basic. It doesn't tell you much else. There are also liquid test kits you use by taking a sample of the solution in a test tube. You measure the pH by adding a droplet of the indicator solution to the water. After mixing it, you will have a color that can be measured using a chart to get a fairly accurate pH level.

For very precise measurements of pH, you need to have the ability to titrate your sample. Titration can seem complex, but once you get the hang of it, it is a great way to see the pH of the solution. We'll talk about titration at the end of the chapter.

Acids and Bases

Now you know that a solution with a pH below 7 is acidic, and a pH above 7 is basic, or alkaline. The word _acid_ originated when scientists often chose Latin words for everything. The term _acid_ relates to the Latin word _acere_. Latin-speaking people used this word when they wanted to say _sour_, like sour lemons, which are acidic, by the way.

A basic substance will feel very slippery and will taste bitter. When bases are dissolved in water, there are more hydroxide ions in the water than there are hydronium ions. Later on, we'll talk about what happens when you put an acid and a base together in the same solution.

When we talk about a solution being acidic, does this mean that there is only an acid in the solution? Not really, all it means is that there is more acid in the solution than there is an alkaline substance. Acids and bases are part of our everyday life. You encounter acids and bases all the time. Most of them are things you might recognize:

Strong and weak acids:

- Battery acid – pH less than 1
- Stomach acid – pH of 1.0 to 1.5
- Vinegar – pH 2.5
- Orange juice – pH 3.3 to 4.2
- Coffee – pH 5.0

Neutral Substances:

These include things like milk (very mild acid) and seawater (very mild base).

Strong and Weak Bases:

- Ammonia – pH of 11.0 to 11.5
- Bleach – pH of 12.5
- Lye – pH of 13.0 to 13.6

Acids and bases have different definitions than you would think. The obvious answer would be that acids give off a hydrogen ion and bases give off a hydroxide ion. This is true of some acids and bases but not all of them. It turns out that, as acids and bases were discovered and figured out, the definition needed to expand. Now, there are several definitions, including the Arrhenius definition, the Lowry-Bronsted definition, and the Lewis definition. These are the essential definitions you should know:

- **Arrhenius definition** – this definition is what you'd think. An acid generates a hydrogen ion, while a base produces a hydroxide ion when placed in a solution. A good Arrhenius acid is hydrochloric acid (HCl), while a good base is NaOH or sodium hydroxide. We will talk soon about what happens when you mix them together.

arrhenius acids and bases

$$HCl \longrightarrow H^+ + Cl^-$$

acid - forms H^+ in water

$$NaOH \longrightarrow Na^+ + {}^-OH$$

base - forms ^-OH in water

- **Bronsted-Lowry definition** – in this case, an acid is anything that donates a proton, while a base is anything that accepts a proton. This broadens the definition and gets rid of the idea of having hydroxide ions as part of the acid-base interaction. It allows for ammonium ions (NH4+) to donate a proton as an acid, while ammonia (NH3) is a base that accepts the proton.

Bronsted Lowry Theory of Acids and Bases

- an acid is a proton (hydrogen ion) **donor**
- a base is a proton (hydrogen ion) **acceptor**

base 1   acid 1   acid 2   base 2

co-ordinate bond

- $H_2O + HCl \longrightarrow H_3O^+ + Cl^-$

- **Lewis definition** – this is a definition that eliminates any protons or ions but strictly involves electron pairs. Acids accept electron pairs, and bases donate them. This means you can have an acid or base that does not have any hydrogen in it. Now you can open up the world entirely to a lot of Lewis acids, such as BF_3, $Fe^{2=}$, and Cu^{2+}. A Lewis base could be NH_3, $F-$, and even ethylene (C_2H_4). When they combine, they can form a covalent bond with one another, which is called an acid-base adduct.

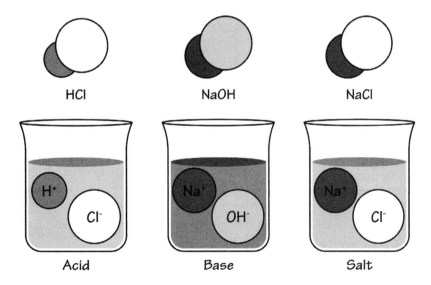

The best way to see what can happen when acids and bases combine in solution is to look at an Arrhenius acid and base in the same solution. Let's try hydrochloric acid and sodium hydroxide. The basic reaction would be HCl + NaOH → NaCl + H2O. Basically, the two substances together make salt and water.

The reaction isn't as simple with other types of acids; remember that Lewis acids and bases can make covalent bonds in *adducts*, but you get the idea. If everything in the above reaction worked out, so all acids and bases were matched mole for mole, the resultant salt solution would be neutral (neither acidic nor basic).

Buffers and Titrations

Buffers are acids or bases that are able to help a solution resist any change in pH. Most are mild acids or bases that will ultimately be able to switch toward being closer to neutral, but it takes some effort to do so. Buffers are great for chemical reactions inside the human body because your body's reactions need a very specific pH range. If you go outside of that range, enzymatic reactions inside the cells do not work well. This is why buffers are nice. You can use them in chemistry experiments as well.

A buffer is a combination of either a weak acid and its conjugate (matching) base or a weak base and its conjugate (matching) acid. Acetic acid is a nice buffer. It looks like this as a matched set with its conjugate base:

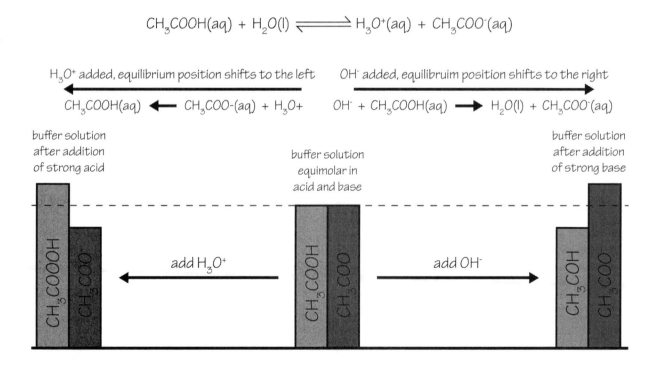

$$CH_3COOH(aq) + H_2O(l) \rightleftharpoons H_3O^+(aq) + CH_3COO^-(aq)$$

H_3O^+ added, equilibrium position shifts to the left OH^- added, equilibruim position shifts to the right

$$CH_3COOH(aq) \longleftarrow CH_3COO^-(aq) + H_3O^+ \qquad OH^- + CH_3COOH(aq) \longrightarrow H_2O(l) + CH_3COO^-(aq)$$

buffer solution
after addition
of strong acid

buffer solution
equimolar in
acid and base

buffer solution
after addition
of strong base

CH_3COOOH   CH_3COO^-   add H_3O^+   CH_3COOH   CH_3COO^-   add OH^-   CH_3COH   CH_3COO^-

You can see by this image that this weak acid is relatively resistant to pH changes, shifting the concentration of CH3COOH and the conjugate acid CH3COO-.

How does a buffer work?

It is the equilibrium between the conjugate acid and conjugate base in high enough amounts and in good balance that keeps the pH relatively stable. In order to decide if a buffer is going to be a good one, you need to know what the concepts of pKa and pKb mean. These tell you a lot about any acid or base.

The terms Ka and pKa are important to acids, while the terms Kb and pKb are important to bases. The ionization constants are called the Ka and Kb. They say how much an acid or base will separate in order to have its different components, such as NaOH versus Na+ and OH- or HCl versus H+ and Cl-. This process is known as ionization.

There is an ionization constant or Kw for water. You derive this from the equation shown:

$$Kw = \frac{[H+]\{OH-]}{[H2O]}$$

If you figured this out, you would get a Kw of 1 x 10^{-14}. The negative log of this would be 14. In neutral water, you would have a natural split of hydrogen ions and hydroxyl (OH-) ions. You need to know that at any time, the Kw = Kb + Ka. If you take the negative log of each of these, you get 14 = pOH + pH. Great! You already know that, so it makes sense so far. Remember that all K values (ka, Kb, and Kw) are in moles per liter, but the pH and pOH values have no units.

Now, to get acids and bases to dissociate in water, you get these equations for an acid (called HA) and a base (called BOH).

HA + H2O ⇆ A- (dissociated acid ion) + H3O+ (hydronium ion)

BOH + H2O ⇆ B+ (dissociated base ion) + OH- (hydroxyl ion) + H2O (the water cancels out)

To get the Ka for an acid, you need to get the molar concentrations of the different substances and figure these out. This leads to this:

$$Ka = \frac{[H+][A-]}{[HA]}$$

A high Ka value means the acid is very strong; it dissociates to a great degree, so the top numbers will be large compared to the bottom numbers. Small Ka values mean the acid is weak and probably makes a great buffer. The dissociated form and the whole form of the acid will be in high numbers. A Ka for a weak acid will be between 10^{-2} and 10^{-14}.

The Kb works the same way, where the Kb = [B+][OH-}/BOH]. The negative log of the Kb is the pkb. Higher numbers also mean a strong base that dissociates greatly. The pKa and pKb together will always be 14.

This is a good time to talk about the _Henderson-Hasselbalch equation,_ a very famous biological and chemical equation. It allows you to test the pH of any buffer solution and will help you find the pH at equilibrium in any acid-base reaction. You can also figure out the concentration of any acids or bases in a solution. The Henderson-Hasselbalch equation looks like this:

$$pH = pKa + \log ([A-]/[HA])$$

This value is used when the concentrations of the different substances are in moles per liter. The pOH is calculated the same way:

$$pOH = pKb + \log ([HB+]/[B])$$

Let's say you want to put this to work by figuring out the pH of a buffer solution of CH3COOH (acetic acid). You know that the acetic acid concentration is 0.2 moles/liter and that the concentration of the conjugate base (CH3COO-) is 0.5 moles/liter. The Ka for acetic acid is 1.8 X 10^{-5}

If you solve for the pH using the negative logs of each, you get this:

$$pH = 4.7 + \log ([A-]/HA]) \text{ or } 4.7 + \log(2.5) = 4.7 + 0.40 = 5.1$$

This means that, at equilibrium, the pH of a solution of acetic acid is 5.1. This is called the acid dissociation constant. It has no real units of value.

You can also use the Henderson-Hasselbach equation to find out how much acetic acid and sodium acetate (its conjugate base) you would need to add in order to make a buffer solution that has the pH you are looking for. You know the pH you want and the pKa (which is 4.7) to get the fraction of sodium acetate and acetic acid you need.

Buffers work within a certain range, so you need to pick the buffer that works best for what you need. There are tables you can use in order to determine which buffer to add to your chemical reaction in order to choose the one that will keep the pH the same while you are running your experiment.

Titration

Titration is a way you can figure out how much of an acidic or basic solution you have. In order to check an acid concentration, you would take your aqueous substance and add enough of a base (little by little) in order to determine when the solution is neutral. Once it reaches neutral, you know that you have added the exact molar amount of base to neutralize the molar amount of acid you have.

How do you do a titration experiment? You simply take a known amount of the solution you are analyzing (be specific about the amount). Set it under a buret and add an indicator that will change color if the solution goes from acidic to basic. It will happen quite quickly once you add the basic solution bit by bit. This is what it would look like:

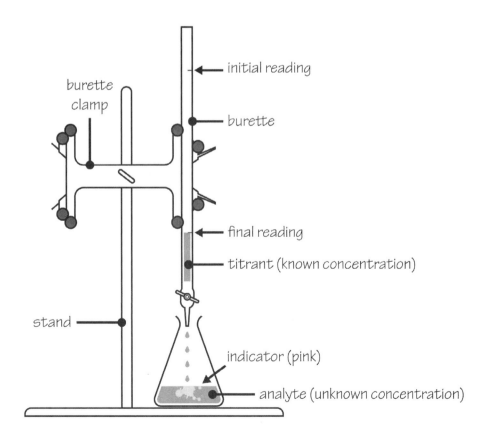

So, once you find the exact amount and the exact number of moles of the base you added to the acidic solution, you will be able to take that mole number and backtrack to find the number of moles per liter (or whatever you want to find out, including the concentration in grams per milliliter if you know the molecular weight of the acid).

As mentioned, the change from acidic to basic (and vice versa) with titration happens quite quickly. You can actually get a titration curve showing how this works. The equivalence point is shown when the precise amount of base has been added:

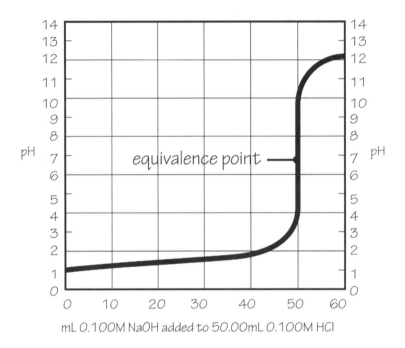

mL 0.100M NaOH added to 50.00mL 0.100M HCl

The trick is to find an indicator solution that will change color near the equivalence point. The equivalence point is when there are equal amounts of acid and base in the solution. It needs to be an indicator that changes color, depending on the pH.

You can do all types of titrations, including redox titrations, precipitation titrations, and complex-formation titrations. Acid-base titrations were just described. Precipitation titrations are done by titrating something with another thing that will precipitate out of the solution at a certain point. The endpoint is reached when you see the precipitate form or if you use an indicator that mixes with an end product to make a colored precipitate.

You could have a situation with a diprotic acid, where it actually has two hydrogen atoms to get rid of. In such a situation, your titration curve would be interesting. You would see a double curve where the two different acidic parts of the same molecule have their hydrogen ion taken off.

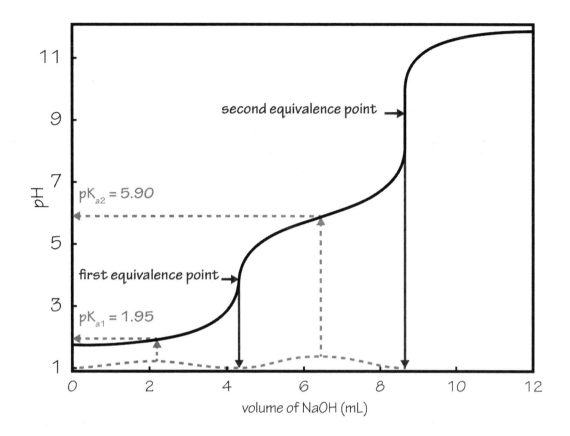

titration diagram for a diprotic acid

Note that the pKa levels of the two different acidic parts of the molecule can be determined by figuring out the point in between the equivalence points, where the curve is the flattest.

Let's Wrap This Up

Acid-base chemistry is an important part of understanding this branch of science. The term pH is simply a handy way of presenting information on the concentration of hydrogen ions in the solution. You should remember that the pH scale runs from 0 to 14 but that it is possible to have numbers off this grid. You should also remember that the pH and the pOH add to 14.

Buffers are weak acids or bases used to keep the pH of a system within a reasonable range when you want to have a reaction happen with few pH changes. You should know what the pKa and pKb stand for in terms of acids and bases. Titrations are used to determine how much of something you have by using indicators and a buret to gradually add one substance to an unknown quantity, awaiting a change to tell you when the equivalence point has been reached.

SECTION 8:
ORGANIC CHEMISTRY

Whether you know it or not, organic chemistry is a constant part of your everyday life. The gas you put in your car is an organic substance. Organic substances are used in industries that make nearly every product you use. In the human body, the top three elements are hydrogen, oxygen, and carbon, so you know that organic molecules are part of the mix.

Organic chemistry is the study of molecules with a carbon backbone. There are zillions of these organic molecules in nature, even though most are made from just carbon and hydrogen, sprinkled with things like nitrogen, oxygen, and even halides like bromine or chlorine.

There are three things you need to take away most from these chapters on hydrocarbons, alcohols, aromatic compounds, aldehydes, and more. These are nomenclature, nomenclature, and nomenclature. What this means is that there are so many different compounds that being able to identify them by name can be really confusing. If you can at least be able to say what something is by looking at it, you will have learned a lot and will be able to move on from there.

We will talk about some of the different reactions that happen in organic chemistry, but these are not as important as knowing the nomenclature. Study the reactions in order to see the trends in how these molecules react with other things; once you do this, you will be able to figure out reactions of all kinds among the many organic molecules you will encounter.

CHAPTER 15:

HYDROCARBONS

You know hydrocarbons well already. These are things like propane, methane, and the many related molecules you see in oil and gasoline. Waxes, asphalts, oils, plastics, and cosmetics are all made from hydrocarbons. They are almost always just made from different lengths of carbon chains attached to hydrogen atoms. Some have every available carbon *spot* attached to a hydrogen atom with no double bonds; others will have double or triple bonds between carbon atoms, so there are fewer available free electrons to pair with hydrogen molecules.

Types and Properties

Hydrocarbons are considered your *basic* organic molecules because they are simple and generally linear. You will name them according to the length of the carbon chain and the number of double or triple bonds in the carbon chain. Just remember: hydrocarbon = carbon + hydrogen. There are four types of hydrocarbons: alkanes, alkenes, and alkynes are covered in this chapter, while aromatic hydrocarbons will be in the next chapter.

Alkanes are simple. If a molecule has no double bonds and is just a chain of carbon atoms with hydrogen atoms at every *free* spot, it's an alkane. Hydrogen attaches to one carbon atom, while carbon atoms can attach to another carbon atom or to hydrogen. The basic chemical formula is C_nH_{2n+2}.

The simplest one is methane. The chemical formula is CH_4, which fits with the basic rules. As you go higher in the number of carbon atoms, the rules will be the same, but the names will reflect the higher number of carbon atoms. There are some general rules to follow, but the rest is pretty basic. Bear in mind that hydrocarbons do not have to be in one long chain but, in order to name them, you need to know how to name each chain. Look for odd passengers, such as chlorine, bromine, or even hydroxide (OH-).

You may know some of the alkanes under more common names; however, you should stick as much as possible to the IUPAC nomenclature (remember that IUPAC means the International Union of Pure and Applied Chemistry). These are the basic rules:

Rule 1: Always find the longest chain. This is the parent chain. You will use this as the main name of the alkane.

Rule 2: Use this table to name your parent chain:

Carbon Atoms	Name	Carbon Atoms	Name
1	Methane	11	Undecane
2	Ethane	12	Dodecane
3	Propane	13	Tridecane
4	Butane	14	Tetradecane
5	Pentane	15	Pentadecane
6	Hexane	16	Hexadecane
7	Heptane	17	Heptadecane
8	Octane	18	Octadecane
9	Nonane	19	Nonadecane
10	Decane	20	Icosane

Step 3: Look for the side chains and name them according to the number of carbon atoms on them. Some will not be carbon chains but will be things like chlorine, bromine, or a hydroxyl ion. These are called substituent groups.

Step 4: You will then number the carbon atoms of the parent chain, with the lowest number being nearest to the carbon atom with any side chain on it. The idea is to have the lowest possible numbers linked to the side chains. This is an example:

The first one is correct because it gives the chlorine substituent the lowest possible number. If you have two possible choices (as with an identical substituent in the same side chains), check to make sure that the lowest possible numbers are assigned to as many of the different side chains on the parent chain as you can. Write the possible choices first, then choose the one where the side chains have the lowest numbers.

Step 5: When you write the name, the parent chain is the last part of the name. Every other substituent is written with the number of the parent carbon chain listed before the substituent name. If there are two of the same substituents, you can use the prefix di- before the name. This is an example:

Here is another one:

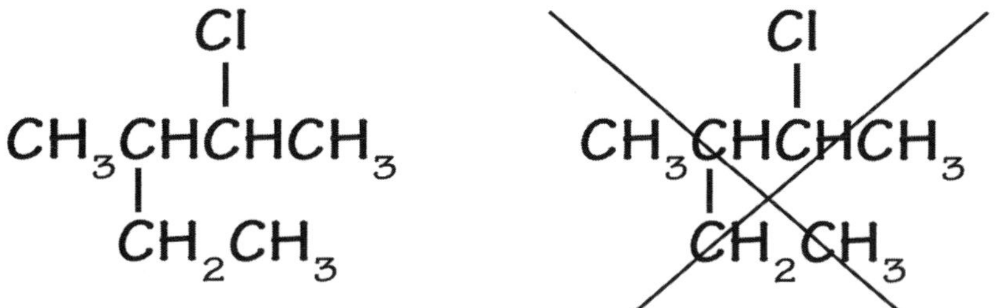

$$CH_3\overset{\overset{\displaystyle Cl}{|}}{C}H\overset{\overset{\displaystyle }{|}}{C}HCH_3$$
$$\overset{\displaystyle }{\underset{\displaystyle CH_2CH_3}{|}}$$

2-chloro, 3-methylpentane

Correct

2-ethyl, 3-chlorobutane

Incorrect

This is tricky because you really need to hunt for the longest chain. If you start on the right and then count carbon atoms to the longest chain, you get a pentane parent chain and then the two substituent chains that come out of that parent chain.

Step 6: Put the substituent chains in alphabetical order and not the order they come on the chain. An example is this molecule, called 5-chloro-2 hydroxy-4-propylpentane:

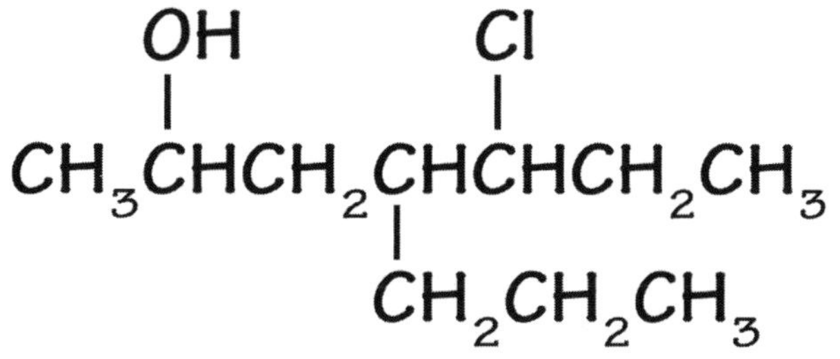

$$CH_3CHCH_2CHCHCH_2CH_3$$
with OH above C2, Cl above C5, and $CH_2CH_2CH_3$ below.

If something is made from just hydrogen and carbon atoms, you can simply write it shorthand as shown in this example:

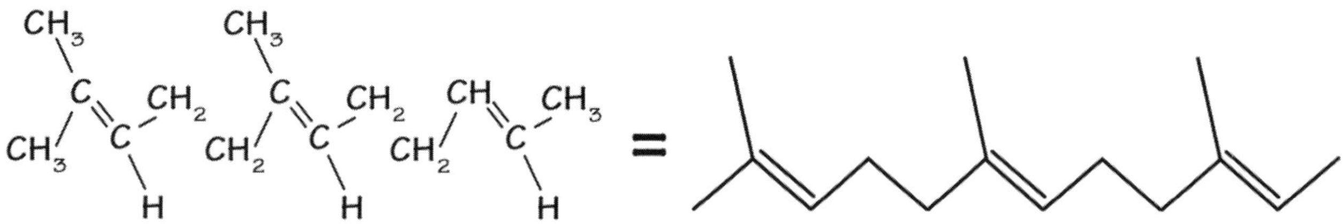

Alkenes and Alkynes

These are unsaturated hydrocarbons with double or triple bonds between the different carbon atoms. A carbon atom with a double bond still has two bonding sites for other things, like hydrogen atoms or a substituent chain containing carbon atoms. This is an example of an *alkene* (containing at least one double bond:

Ethylene

This is called an unsaturated hydrocarbon because it does not have the full complement of sites on each carbon atom. This is because of the double bond between the carbon atoms.

Alkynes have three bonds between two carbon atoms. This allows just one spot for carbon atoms to bind to something besides their neighboring carbon atoms. The triple bond looks like this:

The alkyne in the image is a chlorinated one also attached to an aromatic ring. We will talk about aromatic hydrocarbons in a minute. These alkenes and alkynes are very reactive, so if you mix them with something like bromine, you will easily lose the bond or bonds to make a brominated compound, as shown.

$$CH_3CH=CHCH_3 + Br_2 \longrightarrow CH_3\overset{\displaystyle Br}{\underset{\displaystyle Br}{\overset{|}{\underset{|}{C}H}}}CHCH_3$$

2,3-Dibromobutane

If you run this reaction and mix it with an alkane, nothing will happen. This is because bromine will not easily react with the alkane. If you dissolve bromine in carbon tetrachloride (CCl4), you will get a strong reddish coloration. Add this mixture to an alkene or alkyne, and the bromine coloration will disappear in the solution because it reacts to cause the bromine to disappear. This is called an *addition reaction* involving alkenes or alkynes. Hydrogen bromide will also mix easily with an alkene to make what you'll call an alkyl bromide. This is an example:

$$CH_3CH=CHCH_3 + HBr \longrightarrow CH_3\overset{\displaystyle Br}{\overset{|}{C}H}CH_2CH_3$$

2-butene Hydrogen bromide   *2-Bromobutane*

You can also turn an alkene into an alkane with hydrogen gas. This is also an addition reaction that adds some hydrogen atom to the alkene like this reaction starting with 2-butene and making butane:

$$CH_3CH=CHCH_3 + H_2 \overset{Pt}{\longrightarrow} CH_3CH_2CH_2CH_3$$

The term *Pt* on the arrow means that platinum is needed in the reaction to help catalyze this reaction (get it going). If you do the same thing with water but use sulfuric acid as a catalyst, you will be able to add the hydrogen ion and the hydroxyl ion to make an alcohol like this:

$$CH_3CH=CHCH_3 + H_2O \xrightarrow{H_2SO_4} CH_3\overset{\displaystyle OH}{\overset{\displaystyle |}{C}}HCH_2CH_3$$

If you want to name complex molecules that are alkenes or alkynes, you will need to number where the bonds are located. Use this image as an example:

Alkenes and Alkynes

for an alkene, the prefix is "-en" and the suffix is "ene"

$$\overset{5}{C}H_2=\overset{4}{C}H-\overset{3}{C}H_2-\overset{2}{C}H_2-\overset{1}{C}H_2OH$$

pent-4-en-1-ol
(OH has higher priority than alkene)

$$\overset{1}{C}H_2=\overset{2}{C}H-\overset{3}{C}H_2-\overset{4}{C}H_2-\overset{5}{C}H_3$$

pent-1-ene

For an alkyne, the prefix is "-yn" and the suffix is "yne"

$$\overset{4}{H_3C}-\overset{3}{C}=\overset{2}{C}-\overset{1}{C}H_2-NH_2$$

but-2-yn-1-amine

$$\overset{1}{H_3C}-\overset{2}{C}=\overset{3}{C}-\overset{4}{C}H_2-\overset{5}{C}H_3$$

pent-2-yne

Start the carbon atom numbering at the highest priority end (the amine or alcohol end in these cases). Then label the double or triple bond by the carbon number where you first see the bond located, even though the bonds span two carbon atoms each time.

Let's Wrap This Up

Hydrocarbons traditionally are made from just hydrogen and carbon atoms, although there are hangers-on at times, such as chlorine, bromine, fluorine, and hydroxyl ions. These are found in lots of well-known products, like perfumes, cleaning supplies, gasoline, and oils.

The most saturated hydrocarbon in a line is called an alkane. They are named for up to 20 carbon atoms in a row. You should know those names. You should practice naming those that have side-chains. These can be tricky because you have to find the longest chain of carbon atoms in a row to be able to name these.

Alkenes have double bonds, while alkynes have triple bonds in them. These are more reactive than alkanes and often are used to make brominated or chlorinated alkanes by adding bromine or chlorine to one or both of the double-bonded or triple-bonded carbon atoms.

CHAPTER 16:

ALCOHOLS

An alcohol is easy to remember. If it has a hydroxyl (OH-) ion attached to it, it will be called a *polyol* if there is more than one hydroxyl group associated with the molecule. The alcohol you probably know best is called ethanol or ethyl alcohol. Its molecular makeup is CH_3CH_2OH. There is also methanol or CH_3OH, plus others you may or may not know. Alcohols can be very complex, and because of the hydroxyl group, they are not as oily and sometimes mix nicely with water (as is true of most of the small alcohols).

Types and Properties

It would be easy to say, "just look for the hydroxyl group," except that there are a few rules attached to the definition of an alcohol in chemistry. In order for a molecule to be considered an alcohol, it must be linked to a carbon atom that is already completely saturated with three other ions. The general formula is $C(n)H(2n +1)OH$.

- A primary alcohol is one with this formula: RCH_2OH (at least 2 hydrogen atoms on the adjacent carbon atom).
- A secondary alcohol is one with this formula: R_2CHOH (just one other hydrogen atom on the adjacent carbon atom).
- A tertiary alcohol is one with this formula; R_3COH (no hydrogen atoms on the adjacent carbon atom).

All names ending in -ol mean alcohol, according to the IUPAC chemical naming convention. This is only if there is no other name that takes precedence. If there is a name that takes precedence, you would call the substance *hydroxy-something* to indicate the fact that the hydroxyl group is present. Sugars are the exception. These are polyols, but you wouldn't know it by the name of them.

Ethyl alcohol is named by using the ethyl name to indicate 2 carbon atoms; then just add the -ol to the end of it, indicating its *ethanol*. You couldn't use this for a propane sugar because you wouldn't know where to indicate the difference between a hydroxyl group on carbons 1 or 2. In such cases, you have several options:

1-propanol

2-propanol
or isopropyl alcohol

You see how 2-propanol also goes by the common name of isopropyl alcohol? This is one example of how common names can be confusing as they don't match the IUPAC names. One special example is the OH side chain attached to a benzene (aromatic) ring. It is called a phenol and looks like this:

OH   or   OH

There are other common names to consider. These are things like *wood alcohol*, which is methanol, *rubbing alcohol*, which is isopropyl alcohol, and *propylene glycol*, which is propane-1, 2-diol. There are many polyols you eat all the time. These are sweeteners, like xylitol, sorbitol, and erythritol. Mannitol is used in medicine, but its IUPAC name is hexane 1,2,3,4,4,6-hexol. It looks like this:

Reactions involving Alcohols

Alcohols are easily made from other organic molecules. They are also good intermediates for making other organic molecules. Alcohols can be used to make a lot of things, undergoing dehydration reactions, oxidation, substitution reactions, and esterification reactions. Let's see what some of these look like:

Oxidation Reactions

When you are talking about oxidation in alcohols, you almost always mean a hydrogen atom is lost in the process. Alcohols turn into things like *aldehydes, ketones,* and *carboxylic acids.* They can go further to make even more oxidized things, such as in esterification processes.

Note that you cannot oxidize tertiary alcohols without breaking carbon-carbon bonds; doing so is very difficult, so you can't do anything under normal circumstances. You can double-oxidize primary alcohols, first to get an aldehyde and then to get a carboxylic acid. Secondary alcohols can only oxidize to make ketones.

Oxidation in your Body

Oxidation happens when you drink ethanol (alcohol), which is actually poisonous to you. Animals often drink alcohol when they accidentally eat fermented foods. They have a detoxifying liver enzyme called alcohol dehydrogenase, which removes the oxidated substance to make an acetaldehyde and then acetic acid. Humans have this too, but in varying degrees, depending on the person. Acetic acid is vinegar that can be gotten rid of easily. Ethanol in humans makes acetate, which isn't dangerous.

Methanol, on the other hand, makes formaldehyde (embalming fluid) and formic acid, which are toxic to drink accidentally. Ethylene glycol is the same thing as antifreeze for your cars. It is sweet-tasting, so animals or children will eat it. When this happens, it turns into oxalic acid, which is toxic to your system. All of these toxic byproducts contribute to many accidental human and animal deaths. This is what ethanol and methanol turn into:

If someone is toxic because of ethylene glycol or methanol, you can give them a dilute solution of IV ethanol. This keeps the alcohol dehydrogenase busy, so it doesn't turn as much of the toxic alcohol into even more toxic byproducts. The kidneys can excrete both ethylene glycol and methanol unchanged, which will help stave off toxicity through competitive inhibition of the alcohol dehydrogenase enzyme.

Dehydration to Alkenes

You can dehydrate alcohols, making a double-bonded alkene. The hydroxyl group is reactive and will leave the carbon atom. Water is created as a neighboring hydrogen is stripped off to make an alkene that has gotten *dehydrated* or lost a molecule of water. You can warm an alcohol with concentrated sulfuric acid (H_2SO_4), which is a strong dehydrating agent. It looks like this:

Rearrangements in Dehydration of Primary Alcohols

Step1 - Protonation of the hydroxyl group

Step2 - 1,2 shift of β-hydrogen forming a carbocation

Step3 - Removing β-hydrogen to form a π bond

Notice how the hydrogen atom first attaches to the hydroxyl group, leaving what's called a *carbocation* once the water leaves. A carbocation is very reactive and unstable, so in the end, a pi bond is made with an alkene, being much more stable.

You can also get simple alcohols to become ethers through dehydration. It only works well for small alcohols like ethanol and methanol. Also possible is the substitution of the hydroxyl group for a halogen atom, mostly by mixing the acid that has the halide as part of it (like hydrochloric acid). Finally, you can mix alcohols with acids to make ester compounds.

Let's Wrap This Up

Alcohols have one or more hydroxyl groups on them. There are primary, secondary, and tertiary alcohols as well as polyols. Sugars and other non-sugar, sweet-tasting things are often polyols. They may need to be named by normal naming and numbering conventions.

Alcohols can undergo many different reactions, most commonly oxidation, dehydration, and substitution reactions. In the body, alcohols undergo enzymatic changes, leading to toxic byproducts that can be deadly.

CHAPTER 17:

AROMATIC COMPOUNDS

Aromatic compounds are those with a carbon-containing ring of resonance. If you see a ring and there are alternating double and single bonds or a circle in the middle of the ring, this will most likely indicate you've found an aromatic compound. This resonance is the result of pi bonds in the molecule that share electrons between two adjacent bonds. They are called *aromatic* because they had a particular aromatic smell.

Types and Properties

The simplest aromatic compound in organic chemistry is benzene. By being aromatic, it has a lower heat of combustion and a decreased chance of reactivity compared to other organic molecules of the same size and carbon number. You know benzene as C6H6, or by this image:

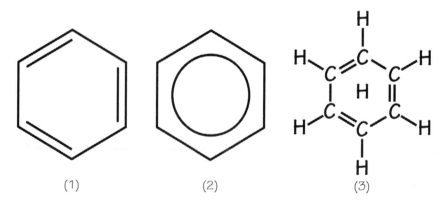

chemical structure of benzene

The circle means the structure is resonant and the double bonds can switch around. What they cannot do, however, is be on adjacent carbon atoms. The double bonds must be separated by a single bond at all times. Resonance means the electrons are *delocalized* and are not stuck within a single bond.

Most aromatic compounds are made by an extraction process with coal tar as the base substance. There are many common names of these compounds, as shown:

Toluene   Phenol   Arisole   Aniline   Benzoic Acid

There are certain naming conventions when there is more than one substituent group on the aromatic ring you should know about. For example, let's say you have a benzene ring with two methyl groups on it. If you study the ring, you can see the two groups can be separated by one, two, or three carbon atoms. You need to name these isomers so you can describe the difference between similar molecules. The terms used are *ortho*, *meta*, and *para*, which help you decide where the substituent groups are located. This image describes what they look like:

Ortho   Meta   Para

These are all called dimethyl benzene but are labeled with the prefixes shown in the image. This way, you can correctly identify the different isomers.

Reactions of Aromatic Compounds

There are ring activators that help the aromatic compounds react in order to substitute or add substituents to the ring. Ring deactivators will do the opposite and make the ring less reactive. Let's look at how you activate a ring.

The best ring activators have at least one set of unshared electron pairs that can stick off of the ring. A hydroxyl group will easily do this (having two unshared pairs on the oxygen molecule). This makes this hydroxyl substituent an activator. The unshared pair essentially hops onto the resonance to create a series of electron shifts that look like this:

These shifts create a negative charge on the ortho or para carbon atoms, where electrons concentrate. After this happens, these carbon atoms are neutrophilic, or areas of *neutrophiles*, that attract any electrophiles in a much stronger way than before. Note that a neutrophile will be negatively charged, while the electrophiles will be positively charged. These images show active rings that are actively searching out something to bind with.

Deactivators are side chains that draw off electrons from the ring, making it less active. These deactivated rings then direct any added side chains to a meta carbon atom instead. A good activator will be at least somewhat positively charged so that electrons from the ring will be *sucked out of the ring* toward the positive charge. The NO2 side group (nitro group) is polar. The oxygen molecules are negative, and the nitrogen is positive. It's the nitrogen that is attached to the ring. This is what draws the electrons from it. The shifting of electrons makes the ortho carbon an electrophile for attaching anything that is neutrophilic onto the ring. It looks like this:

Bromine and other halogens can easily attach to any area that has a slight positive charge. You would use bromine or chlorine gas to provide these halogens. Bromobenzene is a benzene ring with one bromine atom attached to it. The aromaticity of the ring will still be preserved if you add the bromine side chain to it. In this case, bromine is an electrophile (it wants an electron), so, when you mix the dibromine gas with benzene and a *helping molecule* called FeBr3, the ion FeBr4- is created plus a very brief Br+ ion. This is extremely electrophilic and adds to the benzene ring. The process is actually long but looks like this:

Similar reactions can be used to add a nitro group or a sulfonic group (SO3H) to the benzene ring. Each of these involves the shifting of electrons on or off the ring to get the substituent added to the benzene molecule.

Let's Wrap Things Up

Aromatic compounds are those containing the benzene ring, although there are others defined by their strong smell. These tend not to be terribly reactive but are important solvents in organic chemistry. The compounds are resonant, meaning there are delocalized electrons that can travel anywhere on the ring.

Reactions that add a substituent group to the benzene ring do so by drawing an electron away from the ring or by adding an electron back into the ring. The ring can be activated or deactivated by various compounds used to add various substituents to the molecule.

CHAPTER 18:

OTHER TYPES OF

ORGANIC MOLECULES

There are many different molecules called *organic* because they are made mostly of carbon atoms. These include a wide variety of things we will talk about soon, such as carboxylic acids, ketones, aldehydes, and ethers. You should know what these look like and some ways the different molecules are made. You will see how the different organic substances are found everywhere in nature.

Naming Conventions

This might be the place to talk about naming priorities in organic molecules. The naming of many organic molecules gets mucked up by the fact that there are so many side chains involved. There are certain priorities you need to know. If something is an alcohol and a carboxylic acid, for example, you call it a carboxylic acid. There are certain strategies to which you need to pay attention:

From highest to lowest priority, you get this:

group	prefix	suffix
1. carboxylic acid	carboxy-	-carbokylic acid -oic acid
2. sulfonic acid	sulfo-	-sulfonic acid
3. ester	alkoxycarbonyl-	-oate
4. acid halide	halocarbonyl-	-oyl halide
5. amide	carbamoyl- (aminocarbonyl-)	-carboxamide -amide

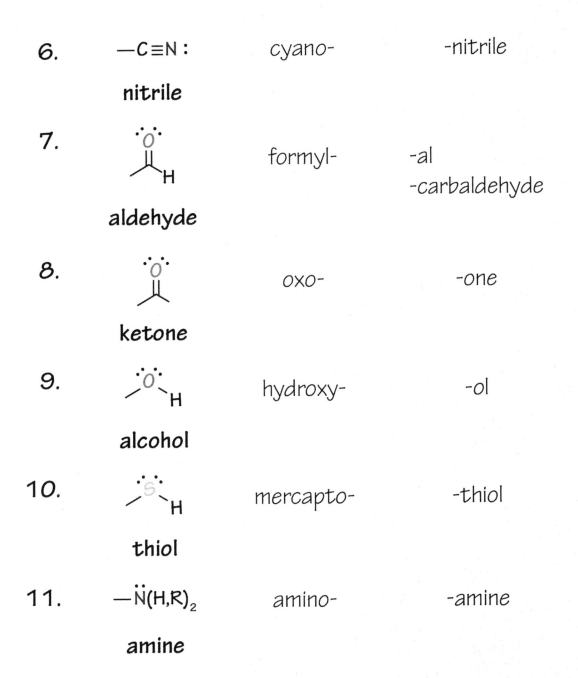

6.	—C≡N:	cyano-	-nitrile
	nitrile		
7.		formyl-	-al
	aldehyde		-carbaldehyde
8.		oxo-	-one
	ketone		
9.		hydroxy-	-ol
	alcohol		
10.		mercapto-	-thiol
	thiol		
11.	—N̈(H,R)₂	amino-	-amine
	amine		

Any alkene plus an alcohol is an *alcohol* with the -ol suffix. You would have something like pent-4-en-1-ol to indicate where the double bond and alcohol side chain are located, respectively.

Certain groups will always be prefixes and not ever suffixes. These are nitro groups, azides, alkoxides, and all halide groups (bromine, fluorine, and chlorine). The will show up alphabetically as you describe the molecule and its side chain as you see here:

Groups That Are AlwaysPrefixes and Ordered Alphabetically

group	prefix	example
—Br	bromo	3-bromopentane
—Cl	chloro	2-chlorohexane
—F	flouro	fluorobenzene
—I	iodo	2-iodobutane
—O-R	alkoxy	methoxyethane
—N$_3$	azido	azidopropane
—NO$_2$	nitro	nitroethane

Ketones

Ketones involve a double-bonded oxygen molecule to a carbon atom. The definition further indicates that the attached carbon atom is also attached to its own carbon atoms (and not to an oxygen or hydrogen atom). This is where you get the R2CO basic formula of these molecules. An easy one to identify is 2-butanone, or methyl ethyl ketone, as shown:

$$
\begin{array}{c}
O \\
\parallel \\
CH_3 - CH_2 - C - CH_3
\end{array}
$$

2-butanone
(methyl ethyl ketone)

When you name these molecules, you will simply say the side chains and then say *ketone*, or you will use the suffix *-one* to indicate that this is a ketone.

Aldehydes

Aldehydes are similar to ketones except that the carbon atom has one R side chain and one hydrogen atom. An example of this is methanal, which you know to be formaldehyde. Ethanal is also called acetaldehyde. Both of these are in this image:

$$
\begin{array}{cc}
O & O \\
\parallel & \parallel \\
H - CH & CH_3 - CH
\end{array}
$$

methanal   *ethanal*
(formaldehyde)   *(acetaldehyde)*

If you are using the IUPAC naming convention, you will use the *-al* suffix to describe this. You will first choose the longest side chain as your parent name (using the same naming convention as in alkane naming). Drop the -e off of the alkane name and add the -al suffix instead. All substituents added are named, with carbon number 1 being the one with the oxygen atom attached to it. This is the <u>carbonyl carbon atom</u>. The carbon atom next to this one is called the alpha carbon, and the one next to this is the beta carbon.

If you have a cyclic or aromatic aldehyde, simply name the ring and add the word carbaldehyde to the ring name. The molecule benzene carboxaldehyde, for example, is this one:

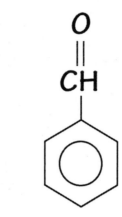

benzenecarbaldehyde

Carboxylic Acids

Carboxylic acids are much more common than you'd think. These are slightly acidic organic compounds where there is a -COOH group attached. As you can figure out, this leaves just one spot for an R chain on the carbonyl carbon atom. This is because it is single-bonded to an -OH side chain and double-bonded to an oxygen atom. These are some examples:

methanoic acid   ethanoic acid   propanoic acid

Look for the -oic acid suffix to define these molecules. Remember that carboxylic acids rank high in the IUPAC naming system; this means you should expect to name something a *carboxylic acid* if you see this side chain.

You will see this in biology and biochemistry all the time. The fatty acids and amino acids in your body are all carboxylic acids. Carboxylic acids are fairly reactive, so you will see them in reactions that make esters, carboxylate salts, amides, and alcohols, among others. This is an example of an amino acid (which also has an amino or NH2 group):

Amino Acid Structure

Carboxylic acids are also good for making the polyester clothing you might wear. The reaction involves mixing a carboxylic acid and an alcohol to get an ester. Many of these together make a polyester substance. Carboxylic acids will help make amides, but usually by first making an ester.

Esters

Esters are organic molecules that have the hydroxyl group on the carbonyl atom of a carboxylic acid replaced by some other side chain, called an alkoxy group. You would call this side chain an -OR group. Glycerides (like the triglycerides in your fat cells) are essentially esters made from a molecule of glycerol. Smaller esters are used to make essential oils or pheromones (these are fragrant). This is an example of a triglyceride ester molecule:

glycerol   3 fatty acid chains

Phosphorus-containing esters are essential parts of the DNA inside all cells. Nitroglycerin is a nitrate ester instead. Most esters in non-biological settings smell sweet or are fragrant in other ways. Esters are used as lubricants for a variety of reasons. If you see the term *synthetic lubricant*, it is probably an ester. The IUPAC name for an ester involves ending the term with the *-oate* suffix. An example is methanoate, which is commonly known as formate. You can simplify the term of an ester by writing this: RCO2R' (indicating two separate R side chains).

Ethers

Ethers are any molecule that goes by the simplified term of ROR', indicating an oxygen molecule between two side chains. These can be cyclic as well. The two R chains can be identical, leading to a symmetric ether; they can also be different, called asymmetric ethers. Diethyl ether is most well known as *ether*, used in medicine as an anesthetic. Glucose and other sugar molecules are essentially ethers in ring form.

The IUPAC name for an ether involves using the generic term *alkoxy alkane*. In other words, the term *methoxyethane* turns out to be CH3-O-CH2CH3 (see the methyl and ethyl side chains?). The longer carbon chain is written last, and the shortest chain has the *oxy* term in it. This is diethyl ether:

Amines

Amines are organic molecules that are derived from ammonia. Remember that ammonia is somewhat alkaline/basic; the same is true of amines. The unshared electron on the nitrogen atom makes it a base. You can have primary, secondary, or tertiary amines, depending on how many carbon atoms are on the nitrogen atom (remember there are three spots available on this molecule). These are the amines you can make with methyl groups:

$$CH_3\overset{\cdot\cdot}{N}H_2$$

1°

methananime
(methylamine)

$$CH_3-\underset{\overset{\cdot\cdot}{}}{\overset{\overset{H}{|}}{N}}-CH_3$$

2°

N-methylmethanamine
(dimethylamine)

$$CH_3-\underset{\overset{\cdot\cdot}{}}{\overset{\overset{CH_3}{|}}{N}}-CH_3$$

3°

N, N-dimethylmethanamine
(trimethylamine}

In the IUPAC naming system, you will choose the longest carbon atom as your parent compound. Instead of the -e at the end of the alkane, you'll add the word -amine. This gives you names like methanamine for the primary amine.

The aromatic amines are different. You name them according to specific parent compounds that are already amines. One of these is called *aniline*. You can substitute one of the hydrogen atoms on the nitrogen group, naming it as shown with this added methyl group:

aniline
(parent)

N-methylaniline
(N-substituted)

Lots of Odd Molecules!

Organic molecules can be very complex. If you think about it, you'd see that much of your body is made from organic molecules. All of human life is based on carbon. There are other organic molecules found in nature. Most essential oils used in medical products and perfumes are organic molecules of some kind. They are extracted from bark, flowers, or other plant parts by steam distillation or boiling. Different molecules will boil off at their own boiling point, leading to the separation of the components. Nonpolar solvents mixed with plant parts can extract out the essential oils too.

Many essential oils are called terpenes or terpenoids. Terpenes have double bonds in them, while terpenoids are similar but have oxygen in them as part of their chemical makeup. Turpentine (not something you'd make perfume out of) is a terpene, while camphor and menthol are some terpenoids. Take a look:

Turpentine   Menthol

Let's Wrap This Up

There are many different kinds of organic molecules, which can get very complicated at times. You should know how to name them according to the IUPAC naming convention. You would need to take an advanced organic chemistry course to see how each of these is made and how they interact/react with one another. Just make sure you recognize them and see how many organic molecules you encounter all the time.

SECTION 9:
BIOCHEMISTRY

In this section, you will put a toehold in the world of biochemistry. Biochemistry, like organic chemistry, could be an entire subject all its own. For the purposes of studying chemistry, however, you simply need to understand the basic components of this vast topic. We will cover the different types of biomolecules involved in living things and talk about enzymology, which is how most chemical reactions happen in nature when biomolecules are involved.

CHAPTER 19:

BIOMOLECULES

There are four main classifications of biomolecules. Of these classes, however, there are thousands of different subtypes of these you will see in living things. Most of your body is made from these molecules (minus water, salts, and mineral compounds). Let's see what these look like:

Carbohydrates

Carbohydrates are sugar molecules. You know the basic ones: lactose (milk sugar), maltose (malt sugar), and sucrose (table sugar). You've probably eaten high-fructose corn syrup (even though it is really bad for your health). Most simple sugars are somewhat sweet; complex sugars are longer-chain sugars found inside your liver as glycogen (strings of glucose molecules) or cellulose (also strings of sugar molecules, but not digestible; this is what makes celery crisp). Let's see the main players:

- **Simple sugars or monosaccharides** – the monomer sugars. A *monomer* is a single unit of something. When you put different monomers together, you get polymers. Many biomolecules are polymers. The main monomer six-carbon sugars are glucose, fructose, and galactose. In nucleic acids, there are two five-carbon simple sugars, ribose, and deoxyribose. These are what they look like:

Monosaccharides

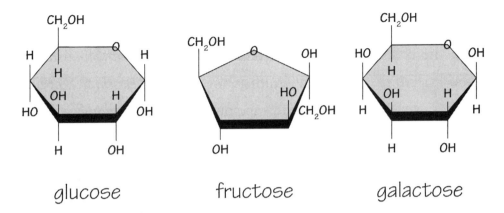

glucose fructose galactose

- **Disaccharides** – the common sugars you probably eat all the time; they are made of two simple sugars linked together. The most common one is sucrose, made when you link glucose and fructose together. You might also call it beet sugar or cane sugar, largely because this is where the molecule comes from. Lactose is milk sugar; it is a combination of galactose and glucose. Maltose is also called molasses sugar; it is a combination of two glucose molecules. Look at the ether bond between the two monosaccharides that make up sucrose.

sucrose

(glucose-fructose)

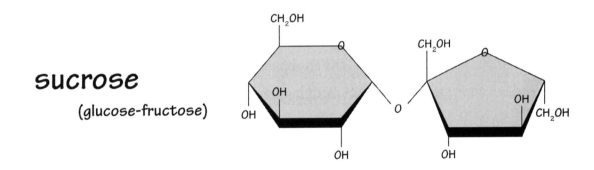

- **Oligosaccharides** – the word *oligo* means *few*; an oligosaccharide is a short-chain polymer carbohydrate made from just a few sugar monomers. An oligosaccharide has three to six monomer sugars linked together.
- **Polysaccharides** – the word *poly* means *many*; a polysaccharide is a long chain of monosaccharide sugars. There are many of these types of molecules seen in nature. In the human liver, the main polysaccharide is glycogen (made only from linked glucose molecules).

In plants, the primary polysaccharide is cellulose, except in starchy vegetables, where the plants build up starch granules; these are also polysaccharides. Amylose and amylopectin are two types of starch. Insects and mushrooms each have chitin as their main cellular polysaccharide. All except chitin are made from glucose molecules in a chain (they differ only in how the glucose molecules are linked together). Chitin is made from a chain of N-acetylglucosamine molecules, which are essentially acetyl amine derivatives of glucose. It's amazing that a shift in glucose linkages affects the properties of these polymers so much.

All of the basic sugars are made only from carbon, hydrogen, and oxygen in a 1:2:1 ratio. Glucose and other simple sugars have the simple formula C6-H12-O2. Glucose is a major energy molecule in the human body; most of the ATP energy used by the cells comes from burning glucose as fuel.

Ribose is one of the few 5-carbon sugars in biochemistry. It is different from the typical 6-carbon sugars we've talked about. Ribose and deoxyribose sugars are used to make DNA and RNA, the nucleic acids of the cells of all living things. You will later see how these sugars are interwoven into the structure of these important biomolecules. Other crucial biomolecules using these sugars are ATP, FAD, and NADH, which are all energy molecules in the cell.

Sugars are considered D-sugars or L-sugars, depending on the position of a certain hydroxyl group. If you look at the second furthest carbon atom from the carboxylic acid carbonyl atom (carbon number 5), the direction it faces by convention will indicate whether it is a D (Dextro) sugar or L (Levo) sugar, as shown:

D-glucose   L-glucose

D sugars and L sugars are enantiomers. These are mirror images but are hard to tell apart unless you use x-ray crystallography to say which is which. In nature, most sugars are called D-sugars. If you ate an L-sugar, you might not taste any sweetness or be able to absorb it because the handedness of a sugar makes a difference in how you perceive or use it. Enzymes have very specific sites used to bind molecules. If the fit isn't right, the enzyme cannot bind to the sugar.

Sugars can be written in ring form or in linear form. They exist in nature as mixtures of these two shapes, often switching back and forth from ring to linear shape. Once they link up to make a disaccharide, the ring shape predominates.

Look back at the molecule of sucrose shown. Both fructose and glucose are 6-carbon sugars, but they differ in how the ring is connected together. Glucose is a hexagonal molecule, called a *pyranose ring*, while fructose is a pentagonal ring, called a *furanose ring*. You can see how the different rings are formed.

Proteins

Proteins are another biomolecule commonly seen in your cells. A single protein chain is called a polypeptide. The monomer unit of all polypeptides is some type of amino acid. There are twenty different amino acids in living systems that mix-and-match to make many different sizes of proteins; however, there are numerous other amino acids that don't ever become part of any protein or polypeptide. The only known elements that make up amino acids are carbon, oxygen, hydrogen, nitrogen, and sometimes sulfur.

Proteins have a number of different roles in nature. Structural proteins for living cells help to make the cell membrane proteins by floating in the lipids that surround each cell. Enzymes are not structural but are *working molecules* that do things chemically inside the cells (see the next chapter). In fact, you can't get much biochemistry done in the human body without using an enzyme to get the job done.

Small peptides, or *oligopeptides*, are used to make neurotransmitters in your nervous system, and amino acids or their derivatives are also used as signaling molecules in the body. Immunoglobulins are large proteins your immune cells make when they make *antibodies* to fight infection. Gluten is a simple protein seen in grains that some people don't tolerate very well.

Amino acids are all unique, but it is only the side chain or R chain that helps the amino acid be unique. This is the basic structure of all amino acids:

Every amino acid has an amine group or NH2 group on one side (which is why they are called *amino* acids; on the other side, they have a carboxyl or -COOH group on the opposite side. The first carbon atom is the carbonyl carbon; next to this atom is the alpha carbon. The alpha-carbon atom is important to amino acids because it always has a side chain called the R side chain. The R side chain determines what amino acid you are dealing with.

Side chains on an amino acid can be as simple as a hydrogen atom, which is the side chain for glycine. Glycine is very simple, while others, like tryptophan, are much more complex. Two amino acids have sulfur as part of the side chain; this is important for the chemistry of the amino acids and the peptide chains they help make. These are the different amino acid classifications:

non-polar	carboxyl	amine	aromatic	hydroxyl	other
alanine	aspartic acid	arginine	phenylalanine	serine	asparagine
glycine	glutamic acid	histidine	tryptophan	threonine	cysteine
isoleucine		lysine	tyrosine	tyrosine	glutamine
leucine					selenocysteine
methionine					pyrrolysine
proline					
valine					

Nonpolar amino acids (tryptophan, phenylalanine, tyrosine, and all true nonpolar amino acids) are hydrophobic (water-hating), so they tend to hide in the interior of proteins or will prefer to coexist with lipids rather than water. These will be the ones that reside inside lipid cell membranes rather than in the watery environment inside and outside the cells.

The carboxyl amino acids have a COOH component to their side chain (and will be acidic amino acids). Amine amino acids (arginine, histidine, and lysine) have a side chain with an NH2 (amine) group on the side chain. These will be alkaline or basic, so they will interact with the acidic amino acids. Aromatic amino acids have an aromatic ring of some kind on their side chain. Other groups include those with hydroxyl groups and *miscellaneous* amino acids, including methionine and cysteine, which have sulfur atoms in their side chains.

When two amino acids combine to begin making a protein, they form a specific chemical bond between the carboxyl group and the amine group. We call this a peptide bond. Many amino acids connected through peptide bonds are called oligopeptides or polypeptides. This is what a peptide bond looks like:

peptide bond

The basic string of amino acids without regard to the actual shape of the protein molecule is called the primary structure of the protein, or peptide. It doesn't end with the string of amino acids, however. Amino acids will interact with one another in specific shapes to create a secondary structure. The two main secondary structures are the alpha helix and beta-pleated sheet. This secondary structure is based on the hydrogen bonding between the different amino acids in the peptide chain. Depending on how the hydrogen bonding occurs, the shape will be different.

Use this image to see what these look like:

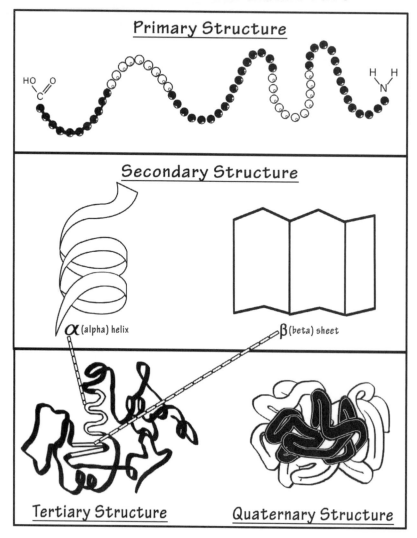

The tertiary structure of any protein involves ways the amino acids interact. Sulfur on some amino acids will form disulfide bridges; nonpolar groups collect in the interior of the protein, while acids and bases attract each other. You can see where this would create numerous 3D protein shapes. When two separate peptide chains attach in semi-permanent ways, this is the quaternary structure. Disulfide bonds between two cysteine or methionine amino acids will be permanent changes to specific segments of the peptide chain.

Lipids

Lipids are the third type of biomolecule seen in living things. These are almost entirely nonpolar and are organic molecules that are carbon-based. In a chemistry lab, these will dissolve in hydrocarbons, such as benzene or an alkane solvent. There are parts of some of these molecules that are polar, but they aren't enough to make these molecules *polar* in any way. There are different types of lipids that vary in structure and function. Let's take a look:

- **Fatty acids** — fatty foods are mostly made from fatty acids. Your body stores fat as fatty acids, or triglycerides, inside the fat cells. These also get broken up to make fuel when sugar/glucose stores are used up. A fatty acid is a long chain of hydrocarbons with a carboxylic acid on the end of it as shown:

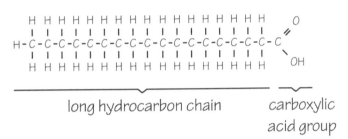

Essential Features of a Fatty Acid

You've probably heard of saturated and unsaturated fats, right? These names essentially refer to the structure of the hydrocarbon chain. A *saturated fatty acid* is one with no double bonds between carbon atoms on the hydrocarbon chain, while *unsaturated fatty acids* have at least one double bond. Polyunsaturated fatty acids have at least two double bonds in any chain.

Fatty acids have common names that aren't important in the span of things but determine which type of oil you are eating or cooking with. There are some called *essential fatty acids* because you need them but can't make them.

Here are a few common ones with differing double bonds on them:

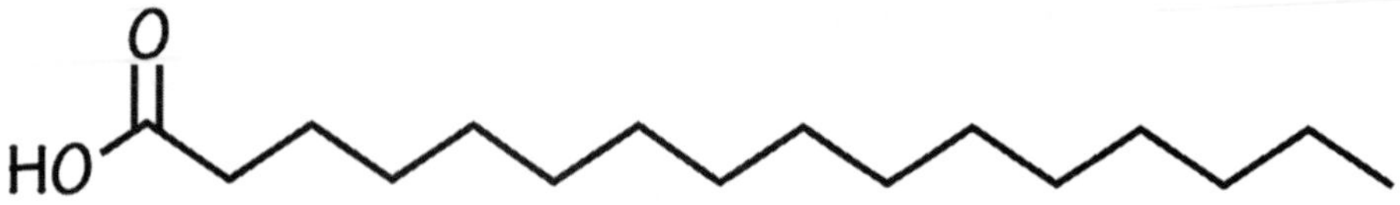

palmitic acid - saturated fatty acid

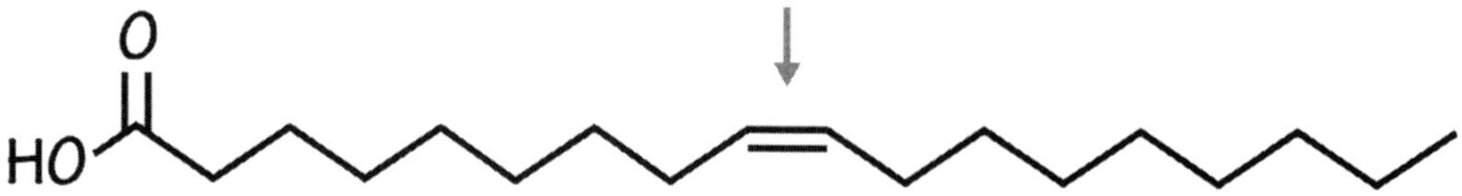

oleric acid - monosaturated fatty acid

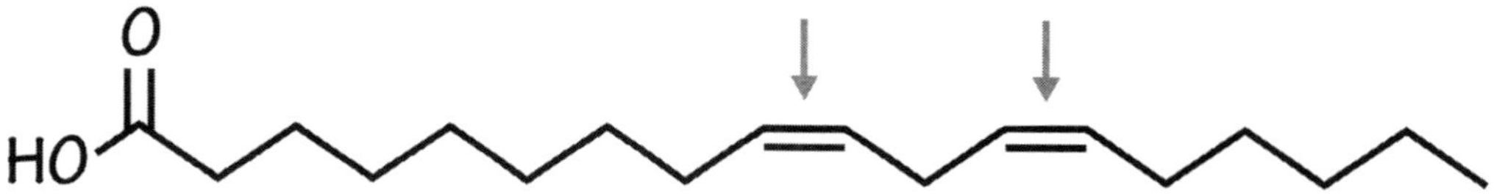

linoleic acid - polyunsaturated fatty acid

The fatty acids with the double-bonded sections shown in the image are *dome-shaped*; these are called cis-fatty acids because the two long chains exit the double bond on the same side. It gives the fatty acid a certain shape. Trans-fatty acids have the side chains exit on the opposite side (trans side) of the double bond. These are relatively straight and more likely to clog things (like your arteries). This is the major difference you see molecularly.

cis-fatty acid

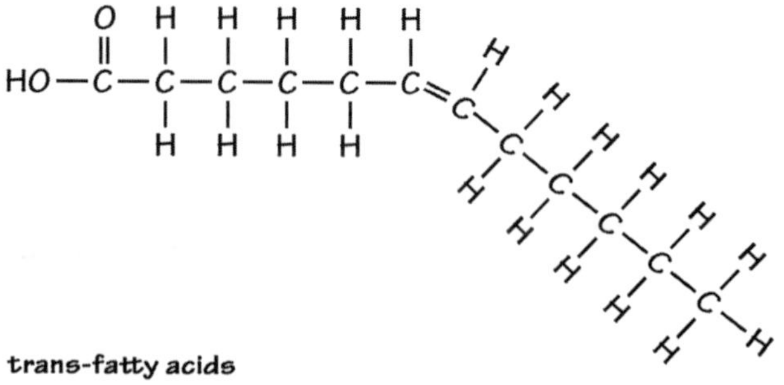

trans-fatty acids

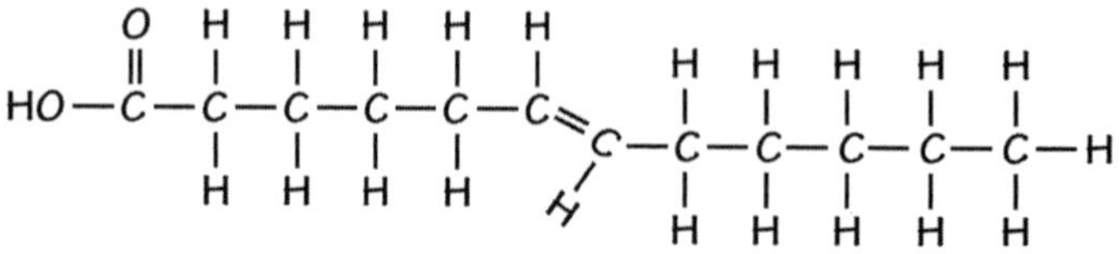

Omega-3 and omega-6 fatty acids are considered very healthy; these are also essential fatty acids. The term *omega* means the last carbon atom. If you count forward (toward the carbonyl carbon) three atoms, you will get a double bond in omega-3 fatty acids. The same thing happens in omega-6 fatty acids, except at the sixth carbon from the end. Two common ones are alpha-linoleic acid and linoleic acid. These can have more than one double bond, but the double bonds at the assigned level (third or sixth carbon from the end) are necessary.

- **Waxes** – there are many different types of waxes. They are malleable solids at room temperature. Those seen in nature include beeswax, the oil in a whale's head, and plant waxes. If you react an alcohol with a fatty acid, you get an ester. Most waxes are esters, as shown in this image:

- **Sterols** – sterols do not look much like the lipids you would normally see, but as they are *opened up*, you would see they are lipophilic and more similar to other lipids. The main characteristic you should know about is the four rings (with different side chains linked to them). This image is characteristic of sterols: they are important to your cells and are basically fatty acids that have folded themselves into a specific series of intertwined rings. Cholesterol is one of the main sterols in your body, often found floating in your cells. The structure looks like this:

Notice the 16 named carbon atoms in three hexagonal and one pentagonal ring. The side chains are very diverse and help make things like cortisol, estrogen, cholesterol, testosterone, etc.

- **Lipid-like Vitamins** – there are four different fat-soluble vitamins necessary for good health, including vitamin A, D, E, and K. Their structures are not necessarily similar, but they do have fat solubility. An example of a fat-soluble vitamin in this image is vitamin A. You can easily see by looking at it that it is fat-soluble:

- **Triglycerides** – these are an example of a nice way to carry fatty acids *in bulk*. They are simply esters made with glycerol and three fatty acids. The fatty acids do not have to be the same. You can have glycerol with only one or two hydroxyl groups taken by a fatty acid, but this isn't terribly common. Here is the basic reaction used to make triglycerides:

glycerol   3 fatty acids   triglyceride
                                         (triester of glycerol)

- **Phospholipids**—phospholipids are fatty acids that have a phosphate molecule (PO_4 $3-$) at one end of the lipid molecule. This is what makes the molecule so polar. The fatty acid chain is still lipophilic, but the end is hydrophilic. This allows the molecule to line up in a sandwich, with the polar ends facing outward and the lipid ends clustered together in their own layer. This is called a bilayer sheet. It makes up the cell membrane of the cells but also can be used in vesicles that transport things. A micelle is a ball of lipids that arrange themselves so the lipids are together, while a reverse micelle is what you'd get if the phospholipid is dissolved in oil. This image helps to explain how this works:

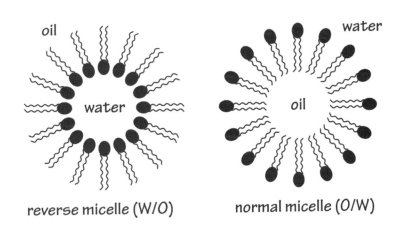

reverse micelle (W/O) normal micelle (O/W)

Nucleic Acids

Nucleic acids are the last type of biomolecule seen in all cells. All genetic material is some type of nucleic acid. The two main types are RNA and DNA. DNA (deoxyribonucleic acid) is usually the stored genetic material inside cells. RNA (ribonucleic acid) has different uses, but the main one is to carry the genetic message in the nucleus to other parts of the cell so that proteins can be made out of the *message* they receive.

Nucleic acids are mostly polymers of nucleotides; the nucleotides are the monomer unit of DNA and RNA. A nucleotide has one nitrogenous base, one pentose 5-carbon sugar, and a phosphate group. The nitrogenous base is unique to the different nucleotides; they help keep two DNA strands together through hydrogen bonding. The phosphate group and alcohol groups on the other parts of the nucleotide are used to connect the monomers together using phosphoester bonds.

nucleotide

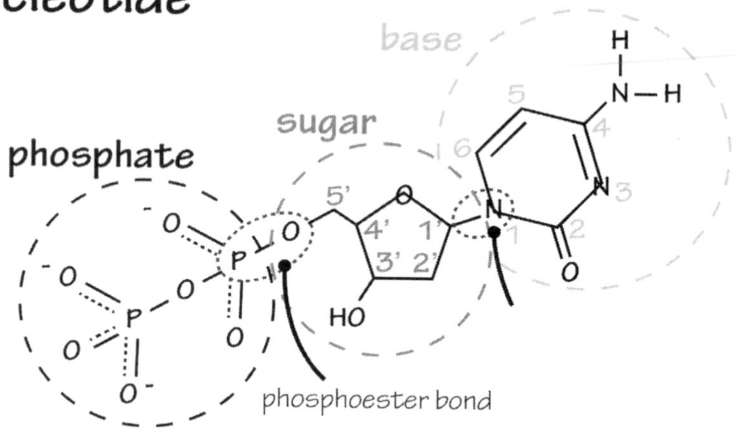

There are five different nitrogenous bases, usually letter-named as A, T, G, C, and U. A stands for adenine, T stands for thymine, and G stands for guanine—you get the idea. When they link through hydrogen bonding, they have specific preferences as to what to bind to. Adenine and thymine like each other; they form bonds to connect, while guanine and cytosine also like each other (in terms of bonding).

The next image shows how DNA fits together. There are the phoshoester bonds used to make the long chain and hydrogen bonds between the nitrogenous bases to make the double-strand. You can also see that the two strands go in opposite directions. The 5' end is the hydroxyl end, and the 3' end is the phosphate end. These strands are called "antiparallel strands."

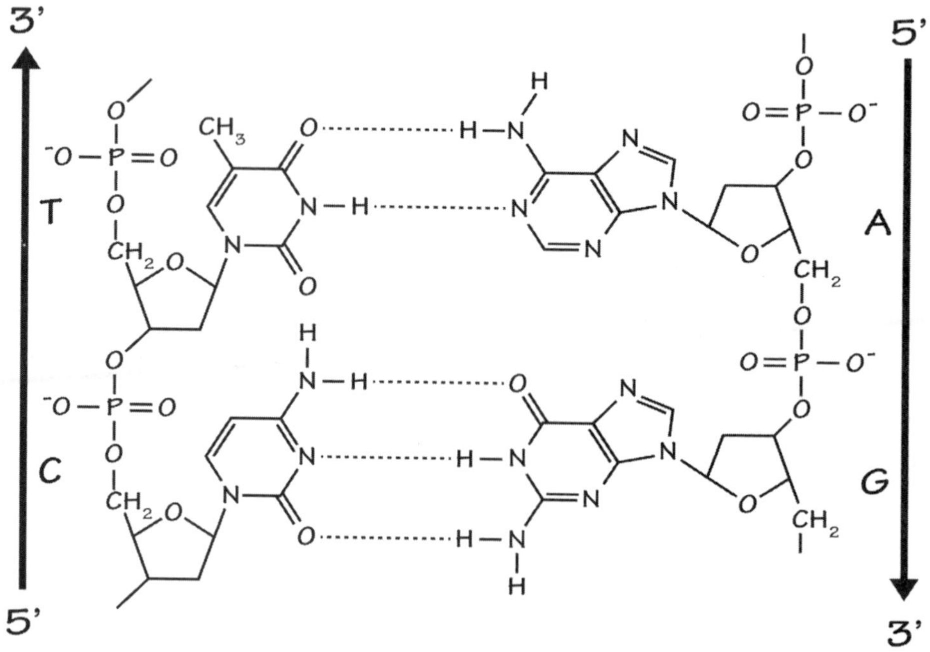

Remember that DNA has deoxyribose as its pentose sugar, and RNA has a ribose sugar. The only difference is that DNA doesn't have a hydroxyl group on the 2nd carbon in the ribose sugar. It turns out that this particular structural change in DNA makes it more stable if the molecule is paired or double-stranded. RNA can be single or double-stranded. There are many types of RNA, including messenger RNA and transfer RNA.

Nucleic acids are a smart idea in nature because, as a polymer, there are countless arrangements. These arrangements help create as many *messages* as necessary to create all of the proteins of life. The DNA essentially tells a story that gets acted out by RNA. RNA goes through many processes to be able to deliver the correct message to the rest of the cell. Once outside of the nucleus, messenger RNA goes to ribosomes, where the message gets *translated* into proteins using the genetic code.

The genetic code is ingenious itself. DNA and RNA are set up as polymers read by the ribosomes in sets of three. Given that DNA has 4 different base pairs in combinations of triplets called codons, you would have a total of 64 separate combinations. Of these, 61 of the combinations make amino acids in a protein chain, while the rest are called START or STOP codons; these help by telling the ribosomes in the cell to begin and end the process of transcription. The process is simplified in this image:

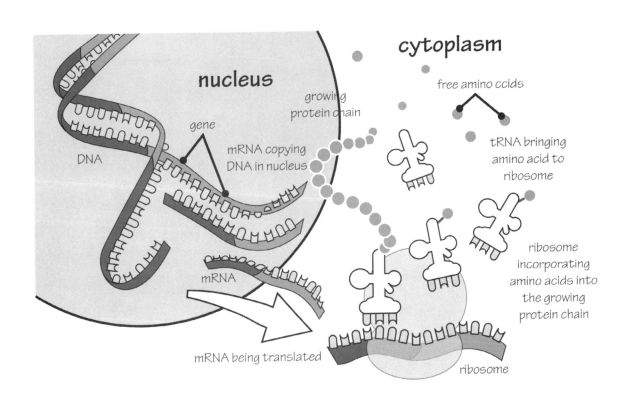

Let's Wrap Things Up

Biomolecules include lipids, carbohydrates, proteins, and nucleic acids. Almost all of these have some type of monomer or single unit that combines to make polymers (long chains). These are all relatively large molecules as well, usually because they are found as polymers more often than as monomers. The variety you get from polymers is wide; this means that they are often unique. The uniqueness in nucleic acids, for example, means that they can send a specific message to ribosomes, which are protein-making factories in the cells.

You should know what the basic monomer structures look like, as well as how they become polymers. Lipids are the most nonpolar of the different biomolecules, except for phospholipids, which have polarity at the phosphate end. Steroids are also lipids, but they look much different from triglycerides. In reality, these are made from triglycerides that twist into the four different rings characteristic of these molecules.

CHAPTER 20:

ENZYMOLOGY

Enzymes are usually proteins that help promote chemical reactions in biological systems. The basic enzyme might take two substrates (beginning molecules), bind to them, then transform them into products (one or two other molecules). The reaction facilitated by enzymes would still happen; the difference is that the enzyme speeds up the reaction manyfold.

Enzymes are called catalysts because they simply speed reactions without getting changed themselves. Once the reaction is complete, the end products fall off, and the enzyme is completely ready to do the same reaction again with more substrates. These molecules have *active sites* so specific for the substrates that they fit like a lock and key system. Once the reaction happens at or near the active site, the products don't fit as well into the active site, so they fall off.

Enzymes do change their shape slightly during the reaction. Basically, they adjust the active site to make the biochemical reaction happen more easily. After the reaction happens, the enzyme might adjust its fit a little bit, allowing the products to fall off. These are not big changes to the enzyme; only tiny configuration changes are made to allow the reaction to happen.

This is an overview of an enzymatic reaction:

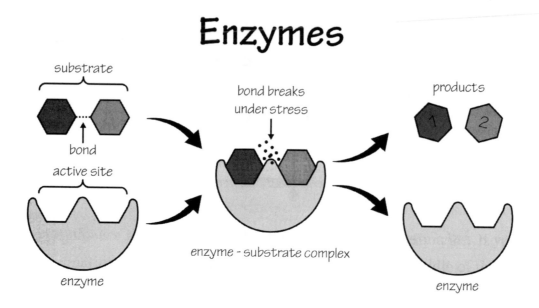

Enzymes

substrate

bond breaks
under stress

products

bond

active site

enzyme - substrate complex

enzyme

enzyme

The reaction would likely happen without the enzyme, but because enzymes put the substrates so close to one another, the reaction is facilitated.

If you look at the whole thing from a thermochemical/energy perspective, you will see exactly why enzymes are so popular in biochemical systems. All reactions have an activation energy, which is a boost in energy necessary to get the reaction going. Even those that are highly energetically favorable (going from a higher energy state to a lower one) need a boost. Enzymes are able to speed reactions simply by reducing the activation energy. This is what it looks like:

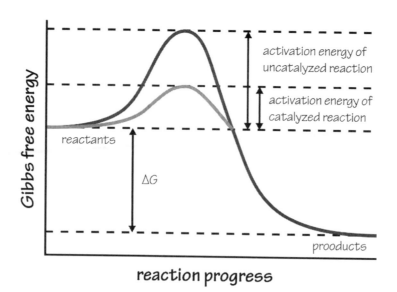

activation energy of
uncatalyzed reaction

activation energy of
catalyzed reaction

reactants

ΔG

prooducts

reaction progress

Gibbs free energy

The reaction shown has a certain energy state. The higher energy is less favorable, which in this reaction means it will give off heat, and the products are favored over the substrates (reactants). The *hump* is lower when enzymes are used, which just makes the reaction speed along more easily.

There is often a middle state in a reaction, where an unstable transition molecule Is made. It is so unstable that it doesn't last long, going to make products as soon as possible. The transition state molecule usually exists at the top of the hump in the reaction shown. Once products are formed, the energy level of the end products is low enough to prevent a reverse reaction from happening.

Even if the products could still go back into reactants, this probably wouldn't happen if there was no enzyme to reverse it. An example of this is the kinase and phosphatase enzymes, which have opposing actions. Kinases put phosphate side chains onto another molecule, while phosphatases remove them. These processes often activate and/or deactivate a certain molecule in the signaling systems of the body. This is how they work (note that the kinase enzyme needs ATP or ADP-P to deliver the phosphate group to the substrate).

Phosphorylation - Dephosphorylation

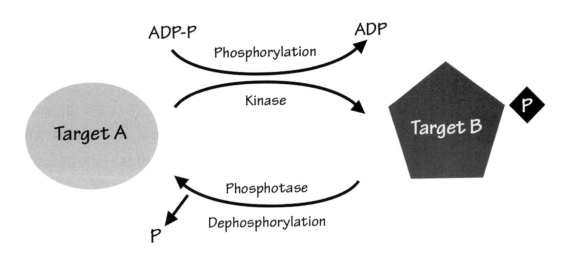

In some systems, the activation energy is provided through the application of heat. When you heat a reaction, you allow energy into the system in order to get the reaction over the hump (activation energy). Enzymes reduce the activation energy rather than provide the energy needed without the enzyme.

Most enzymes are proteins, except in areas of the nucleus and ribosomes. In such systems, there are RNA types called *ribozymes* that actually catalyze reactions. In reality, it doesn't matter what an enzyme is made of. As long as it is large and catalyzes a reaction in a biological system, it is technically an enzyme.

Environment and its Effects on Enzymes

Remember when we talked about the effect of temperature and pH (among other things) and how important they are to the reaction going forth or not? The same is true of enzymes. These are very reactive to the temperature and pH of the environment. Proteins, in general, are delicate molecules. A short exposure to heat or the wrong pH could quickly denature a protein. Denaturation could mean the protein loses its shape or coagulates into a messy ball of amino acids—neither of which leads to a functional protein.

These are the things an enzyme needs to be concerned about:

- **Temperature** – usually, a high temperature spells disaster for any proteinaceous enzyme. Mildly high temperatures, however, could help speed the reaction along. Enzymes have a specific range of tolerability. Outside of the range, the enzyme activity will drop dramatically.

- **pH** – the active site on many enzymes will be either acidic or basic. The pH of the environment affects these sites significantly, making them have higher or lower enzymatic activity. Very high or low pH levels will also denature proteins. This is what happens to the proteins you eat in the low pH (acidic) environment of your stomach. Most enzymes have a specific range they like best.

- **Enzyme and substrate concentrations** – it makes sense that if you have more enzyme molecules in the system, the reaction will go faster. The same thing is true of substrate concentration. On the other hand, if you increase your substrate concentration above a certain level, nothing much will happen because all the enzyme sites have been saturated already. In general, though, more substrate means a faster reaction, as long as you add enough of all the substances you need in the reaction process.

- **Inhibitors** — enzyme inhibition is important in medicine. Enzymes are not perfect and will sometimes be tricked into binding with an imposter. If this happens, the enzyme won't work well unless you add substrate at a high enough concentration to compete with the inhibitor. Noncompetitive inhibition involves a substance that binds away from the active site. It tends to do enough damage to the enzyme or changes its shape, so it doesn't work well, even though the active site is available. This image shows you what these look like:

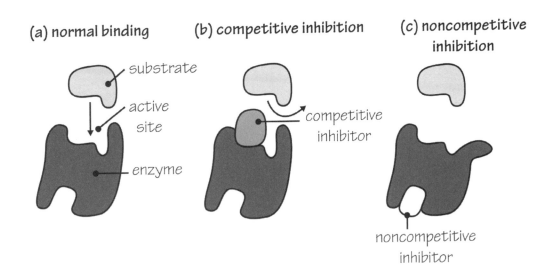

Let's Wrap Things Up!

Enzymes are any molecule that helps catalyze (speed up) a reaction. Most enzymes are proteins, but there are a few ribozymes in nature, made from RNA segments. The enzyme has one or more active sites that allow substrates to bind, giving them a good chance of reacting quickly with one another.

Enzymes reduce the activation energy of a reaction, allowing it to proceed more easily. After the reaction, the products break away, leaving the enzyme ready to work again to facilitate another reaction. Because enzymes are delicate, they are responsive to temperature and pH. Inhibitors will reduce the activity of the enzyme in a couple of different ways.